Lazy Perfection

THE ART OF LOOKING GREAT
WITHOUT REALLY TRYING

By Jenny Patinkin

Running Press
PHILADELPHIA

Published by Running Press,
An Imprint of Perseus Books, LLC,
A Subsidiary of Hachette Book Group, Inc.

Books published by Running Press are available at special discounts for bulk purchases in the
United States by corporations, institutions, and other organizations. For more information,
please contact the Special Markets Department at Perseus Books, 2300 Chestnut Street,
Suite 200, Philadelphia, PA 19103, or call (800) 810-4145, ext. 5000, or e-mail special.
markets@perseusbooks.com.

ISBN 978-0-7624-6144-8
Library of Congress Control Number: 2017931626

E-book ISBN 978-0-7624-6145-5

10 9 8 7 6 5 4 3 2 1
Digit on the right indicates the number of this printing

Cover and interior design by Amanda Richmond
Edited by Jennifer Kasius
Typography: Brandon, Arno, and Dankita

Running Press Book Publishers
2300 Chestnut Street
Philadelphia, PA 19103-4371

Visit us on the web!
www.runningpress.com

For my family who is so precious to me,
Doug, Lila, Phoebe, and Olivia.

You bring me more happiness, gratitude, and joy than even my
most cherished concealer, and that's saying a lot, because I really love
concealer. But I love you all more. Concealer patches me up,
but you fill me up, each and every day. You are the hearts of my heart.

Contents

Introduction

THIS IS A BOOK FOR WOMEN WHO LIKE MAKEUP, BUT DON'T
necessarily like to wear a lot of it. One sentence in and I'm sure you're
already wondering why in the world I've bothered to write a book about
beauty for women who aren't huge makeup wearers, but this is not really a
"makeup book." This is a book about *Lazy Perfection*, and Lazy Perfection
is about how you can put in minimal effort with your beauty routine and
still get results that will make you look and feel lovely. Sure, you probably
enjoy makeup and wear a little of it, or at the very least are intrigued by
it, but if you've picked up a book with the title *Lazy Perfection*, I'd say the
chances are good that you're not operating at YouTube Beauty Guru level,
putting in forty-five minutes on false lashes and contouring every time
you have to leave the house.

I've written this book for women who like makeup, but don't wear a lot
because they don't feel like they know what they are doing, or who have
never really worn makeup, but want to give it a try, or who don't like the
way their makeup looks and want to make some adjustments, or who
want to learn how to streamline their routine so that they can get out the
door faster, looking and feeling great, or who, most of the time, pretty
much just can't be bothered to put any on. This book is about easing the
anxiety that comes with not knowing how to choose the right makeup,
answering the questions you didn't even know you were supposed to ask,
giving you the tips and tricks you had no idea existed, and walking you
through a few simple steps that will put you on the road to a gratifying,
flattering, and stress-free beauty routine.

So, What is Lazy Perfection?

Maybe we should start off by talking about what Lazy Perfection *isn't*. First and foremost, Lazy Perfection isn't about being actually lazy. I hear women talk all the time about the improvements they'd like to make to their appearance—they aren't happy with their skin, they have dark circles, they don't feel like their eyes "pop" . . . but then in the same breath, they tell me that they don't enjoy applying makeup and don't really want to take the time to deal with it. Ladies—you cannot have it both ways. If you want to make an adjustment to your beauty look, some effort will be required. The extent of that effort is up to you. *Lazy* is a totally relative term, but no matter how much time you're willing to put into it, it's going to take a commitment. Five minutes, ten minutes, twenty-five minutes . . . One woman's fast-and-simple is another woman's holy-crap-that's-a-lot-of-effort, so you are the only one who can decide what it means to you.

Secondly, Lazy Perfection is also not about being *perfect*. Perfect is a myth. Very few women have completely symmetrical faces, or features that conform to some unattainable standard of perfection. We are real, human, flesh and blood, some of us with one eye larger than the other or one brow thinner. We can totally enhance or improve our appearances, but true perfection does not exist. Perfection is a reflection of our own personal beauty ideals, our own standards of beauty, so this method should really be called Lazy Whatever-You-Think-Is-Pretty, but the name isn't as catchy.

Get to the Point . . . What is Lazy Perfection?

In my Lazy Perfection approach, I take a holistic overview to beauty. Which means the makeup we use has to work not only with our facial anatomy and coloring (obviously), but also with our personal style, lifestyle, and technical skills. Everything has to be in harmony so that you always look and feel like just a more put together version of you. That's when you'll feel the most confident, natural, and at ease . . . and, in a nutshell, that's Lazy Perfection.

I want the Lazy Perfection girl to always feel like *herself,* not as though she's been given a full *America's Next Top Model* makeover, opening her eyes at the end and being totally flabbergasted. The Lazy Perfection version of "natural" is when you look like you . . . only a bit more polished, refined, and chic . . . no matter how much makeup you are wearing. I can't tell you how many celebrities and social media-ites use makeup to create features on their faces that don't exist in nature, but that's not how I approach beauty. Lazy Perfection ENHANCES what you have; it isn't a do over.

With every client I see, I strive to give them a look that they can easily replicate at home, to set them up for success. If eyeliner is so frustrating for you that you have given up and just don't wear any, I would never suggest an advanced technique like a liquid liner cat eye. That's not Lazy Perfection approved. If you live in yoga pants or jeans and a T-shirt, I am not going to suggest metallic eye shadow and full coverage makeup. That's not in Lazy Perfection harmony. And if you only want a ten-minute makeup routine, I am not going to recommend a fifteen-step makeup program. Because that's not Lazy Perfection, either.

Too often in these days of reality TV and social media, women have a preconceived notion that makeup needs to be totally

TRANSFORMATIONAL and LIFE-ALTERING. I know this isn't going to make me super popular among my retail beauty friends and colleagues whose careers depend on the belief that makeup is terribly important, but really, when you think about it, it's just makeup. What I mean is, if you are sure that the newest eye shadow palette is going to CHANGE YOUR LIFE, or that if only you could find the IDEAL red lipstick or achieve the ULTIMATE cat eye, you'd reach nirvana then Lazy Perfection isn't going to be for you.

Zen and the Art of Lazy Perfection

To be Lazy Perfection, you must first understand that makeup is not the destination, it's the journey. Wow. I'm starting to sound pretty hippie-dippy here, but let me tell you what I mean. Makeup isn't going to alter the path of your destiny, and it's not going to drop luck and eternal joy in your lap. It's not a life raft we have to cling to for our very survival. It's more like a good pair of floaties that can prop you up and make you feel more secure.

What makeup can do for you is bring you feelings of self-confidence and empowerment. It can make you want to make eye contact or smile when you didn't feel good enough to do it before. It can put the spring in your step that comes from feeling great about how you look. And the admiration you get from others can make you feel like the most successful woman in the world.

TPW

That Perfect Woman. Everyone crosses paths with her now and again. She's the girl in high school who was a cheerleader AND valedictorian. She's the full-time working mom who makes homemade cookies and goes to every soccer game. The colleague who kills it in presentations with her clever wit and beautiful smile but still crawls under your desk to help you find your missing earring.

That Perfect Woman always looks terrific. She has lovely skin, beautiful hair, and a wardrobe that's appropriate and chic at all times. She finishes a yoga class looking even lovelier than when she started. Not a blotch, frizz, or a smudge in sight.

Sigh. I know, I know. It's not very "girl power" of me to admit that other women can inspire feelings of inferiority, because we're adults for goodness' sake, and we're supposed to stick together, and support each other, and not compare ourselves, and blah blah blah.

But on days when the giant zit on my chin could launch its own hashtag (#jennysgiantzit) or my hormone-inflamed pores could double as an overhead storage bin, it's hard not to feel a little shaky in the self-esteem department. Those are the times I am in awe of TPW. It's never jealousy or envy. I *admire* her.

So you're probably wondering . . . *How in the world does she do it*? Was she touched by the wand of the Perfection Fairy? Does she have to set her alarm for ridiculously-early-o'clock to get herself ready? Did she whip up a batch of Polyjuice Potion using a strand of Cameron Diaz's hair? None of the above. TPW simply understands how to harness the power of Lazy Perfection. And in this book, I'm going to share with you all the things you can do to make it work for you, too. So let's get ready to saddle up.

Sheriff of Lazy Perfectionville

Bet you're wondering how I earned my Lazy Perfection gold star, so let me give you a little backstory. I have always loved makeup, but I didn't even consider making it a profession until I was almost forty. Look up *late bloomer* in the dictionary. There'll be a picture of me.

In my late twenties, I got married, had kids, and settled into ten years as a stay-at-home mom. I had three daughters in less than four years, so makeup wasn't a big part of my life, to say the least. But when my youngest daughter was in school full-time, I knew I was ready to get back in the workforce.

I was volunteering at my daughters' schools and with other local organizations to keep the bored-mommy-blues at bay when I met a wonderful artist who recognized my raw makeup abilities and encouraged me to do some professional training. That's when it all started to gel. I did my training, and three weeks later I was signed by a huge international artistry agency and jumped right into the industry.

It became clear to me very soon after, that working with models and celebrities wasn't feeding my soul. As much as I love creating beautiful looks on young, unlined, taut faces, it was my friends who really helped me get some clarity on what my next step should be.

They would say to me:

"I never learned how to do my makeup."

"I don't want to wear a lot."

"I hate shopping for makeup."

"My mom didn't wear any makeup, so I never had a role model."

"My face is changing; I need to figure out how to wear more flattering makeup."

"I have no idea what I'm doing, can you show me how?"

It became crystal clear that these women didn't need more makeup; they needed more education. And that's when my Lazy Perfection philosophy came together.

It's what led me to develop my own line of handmade makeup brushes, which are now sold all over the country. It brought me TV appearances and professional beauty expert gigs, which I now travel for all the time, talking about makeup, skincare, and Lazy Perfection; it brought legions of clients to my door asking me to give them the Lazy Perfection Look; and it inspired me to open my Lazy Perfection Beauty School where I teach women in a private setting how to achieve their ideal makeup look.

Getting Schooled

At my beauty school, I work with women of all ages, showing them what I am going to show you here in this book:

- How to clearly identify your beauty intentions and objectives
- How to reduce the clutter in your bathroom and cosmetic case
- How to sync your beauty routine with your lifestyle
- How to identify the beauty looks that will suit your personal style
- How to select the products that flatter your facial anatomy and coloring
- How to stay current with the trends without looking trendy
- How to look youthful and fresh
- How to shop for your makeup without stress, anxiety, or guilt
- And how to do it all efficiently and easily

What I have found in working with my private clients is that MORE WOMEN WANT TO WEAR LESS MAKEUP.

So many women want a simple, clean look, but the beauty industry doesn't focus on them because, well, it's not as lucrative to sell a customer one lipstick when you can sell her a lipstick, a lip liner, *and* a lip gloss. Beauty is a business, after all.

When it comes to makeup and beauty, there's just SO MUCH. So many brands and products, so many ads, so many videos, so many blogs, so many magazines, so many shows. Even as a professional makeup artist, I've been overwhelmed walking into a beauty department or specialty store; my senses so bombarded that I literally have turned around and walked out.

Makeup isn't something we're born knowing. For some women it comes instinctively—for others, not so much. But you *can* learn how to do it. Maybe you won't end up being Monet, but you don't have to be a scribbler for the rest of your life, either. Sure, it requires some practice, but so does cooking, driving, or tying your shoes. Learning how to do anything new takes time.

Like any other education you undertake, it expands your horizons and your choices. Still want to go barefaced? Great. That's your call. Want to bump up your eyeliner one day? You can do that, and do it with confidence. And if you want to have a professional makeup artist apply your face from time to time? That option never has to be taken off the table. The point is, by learning and practicing, you get to take control of how you look, and ultimately of how you feel about yourself. By the time you're done with this book, you are going to be living in TPW's world.

What's the Lazy Perfection Look?

I know lots of you are probably already thinking to yourselves, "Jenny, I am no good at applying my makeup. I am never going to be able to get it right." But I don't want you to listen to that inner voice.

Know why you can do it? Because Lazy Perfection isn't a cookie-cutter, five-minute makeup plan. It's not even a makeover plan at all. It's your guide to discovering what's going to work best and look best on you—you and only you. You can customize it however you want. I'll tell you one thing that's for sure—the Lazy Perfection Look is never, ever overdone, overworked, or heavy-handed.

The Lazy Perfection Look is a whisper, not a shout. It's small details, not grand gestures. And it's about working with your natural features instead of struggling against them.

In learning the Lazy Perfection Look, you'll discover the ways in which smudging softens and enhances the features, small movements give more control in the application than big ones, and how to use less makeup to look fresher and younger.

Lazy Perfection isn't about CHANGING how you look, it's about using subtle details to enhance the loveliest features on your face so that they can be the star of the show, while the rest of your features are a strong supporting cast.

Lazy Perfection Cover Girl

TPW is lovely. It's not just that she's wearing makeup. She's wearing the right makeup. Her clothes don't look great by accident. She knows what colors and styles work for her. And her hair doesn't gleam and bounce the second she rolls out of bed. She chooses the products that are going to give her the best results.

Here's the bottom line. Makeup is wonderful and fun, and it can make us feel confident, empowered, and beautiful. But despite all the messages we get from magazines, movies, television, and one another about how we *should* look, what we *need* to buy, and how we *have* to do it, makeup isn't going to alter who we fundamentally are.

TPW isn't That Perfect Woman because she has pretty hair and clear skin. She's That Perfect Woman because she clearly feels good enough about herself that she doesn't need to make anyone else feel bad. She's secure and happy with how she looks so she can cheer you on until you feel great, too.

I promise you, by the time you're done reading this book and putting my Lazy Perfection methodology into place, you'll be someone's TPW, too.

CHAPTER ONE

The Ghost of Beauty Past

IF I WERE SAYING THIS ALOUD TO YOU, IT WOULD BE IN A SOFT, murmuring, sympathetic tone . . . I know it's hard to clean out your makeup kit. I understand. I truly do. You've got a lot of dollars invested in there, and a lot of really great memories about the time you felt gorgeous in that eye shadow or sexy in that beautiful lipstick. And you think, wow, I should totally keep this because I spent a lot and maybe I will wear it again someday and feel those feelings all over again. I know it can be tough to part with the makeup that makes you sentimental, like a gloss you wore to your wedding, or a foundation that used to make your skin glow.

But part of embracing Lazy Perfection is looking clearly at what works for you *now*, and what simply doesn't suit you anymore. Let go of the guilt, let go of the attachment, and let go of the past. Lazy Perfection is a path to a fresher, more modern beauty routine and your kit, inhabited by the Ghost of Beauty Past, is holding you back.

Give Up the Ghost

We could spend lots of time talking all about the emotional reasons
we buy so many beauty products, like the satisfying impulse purchase
of adorable hot pink makeup brushes or when we got talked into buying
a metallic seafoam-green eye shadow, but the bottom line is, why is
that metallic green eye shadow still in your kit? It's not in fashion and it
doesn't flatter you, so why do you still have it? And those pink makeup
brushes? They shed and feel rough on your skin. You still have them
because why?

Seriously. I've helped clients purge makeup from brands that haven't
existed since the '90s, or lipsticks they wore at their weddings ten years
ago, or, in one instance, an eyeliner that was purchased—no kidding—
in 1979. For a particularly sentimental client, we had her makeup
compacts cleaned and mounted in a shadow box, which she put on
display on a bookshelf.

I'm not trying to makeup shame anyone, but if you are serious about
getting on a Lazy Perfection Track that will streamline your routine
and give you a gratifying and beautiful result, then it's time to clear
the clutter.

Cosmetic Cleanse

The Lazy Perfection Cosmetics Cleanse is a system for really figuring out
what you can live with, what makes you feel good, and what you won't even
miss. It's like finally admitting that you have to clear away the potato chips
and cookies from your pantry and stock it with something that won't give
you heartburn . . . or cellulite.

So how can we look objectively at what needs to be purged? It's tough to step back and assess with brutal honesty what really flatters us and what we really need, but I am going to take you through the process of elimination.

There are three basic reasons to clear your cache of makeup: You have . . .

1) Items that don't look good on you
2) Items that are dirty or broken
3) Items you haven't worn in the past one to two years, or more

You'd think that because buying makeup is such an emotional experience that getting rid of it would be, too, but in my experience with my clients, it's really easy once you start to chuck out the old, in favor of starting fresh. It's cathartic to finally accept that you're never going to wear that frosted green eye shadow again and that you've moved on from the days when Cyndi Lauper was your beauty inspiration. When you get going with my Lazy Perfection method, you'll be thrilled by how easy it is to rid yourself of the things that are just taking up space and haunting you.

Pretty Purification

First, gather all your makeup—from your drawers, counters, cases, office, gym bag, pockets, and the swirling vortexes at the bottoms of your purses—and put it all together in one place, like a basket or a box. This part of the process can yield all sorts of fun rediscoveries, so make sure you are as thorough as possible. You never know what'll turn up in your winter coat pocket or the back of your desk drawer.

Next, find an area with plenty of surface space. I like to do my purges on the dining room table or in the middle of my floor, on top of a couple of old white towels or sheets. That way I can lay everything out side by side in one field of vision and see it all against a bright, clean backdrop.

This is where it starts to get interesting. You'll want to divide everything into groups based on the product category. Here are the most common product categories I see with my clients:

- Primers and eye shadow primers
- Foundations
- Concealers
- Powders
- Bronzers
- Blushes and highlighters
- Eye shadows
- Eyeliners
- Eyebrow pencils/powders, etc.
- Mascaras
- Makeup brushes
- Lip pencils
- Lip glosses
- Lipsticks
- Beauty tools, i.e., eyelash curlers, tweezers, sponges, and powder puffs

JUST STOP allowing cotton buds, cotton balls, stray hairs, pencil shavings, empty sample packets, full sample packets, and old tissues to accumulate in your kit. They get in the way of what you can see and make everything feel dirty. Get in the habit of regularly tossing these disposable items and the samples you'll never use.

Here's what I want you to do now. Group by group, go through each item and ask yourself the first and most important question in the Lazy Perfection Purge process:

When is the last time I used this product?

If it's been more than two years, it automatically earns a place in the trash can. Boom. Just do it. After the first time, you'll like the sense of empowerment so much, every subsequent disposal will give you a rush. Bye-bye, Ghost of Beauty Past. Now, take a look at what's left and ask these questions:

Is this product or container broken, crushed, shattered, or otherwise nonfunctional?

A crushed, crumbly mess of makeup is doing you absolutely no good. You can't transport something with no lid or cap because it'll get all over your other makeup. If your blush or powder is shattered and applies in big, blotchy chunks onto your skin, then trash it! Makeup brushes that shed enough hair to create your own cyborg puppy or that have broken, dented, and misshapen bristles are beyond the point of no return. You have to give them a loving but firm send-off.

> JUST STOP hanging on to eye shadows or powder products where you have "hit pan," i.e., gotten to the very bottom. It won't get picked up evenly by your makeup brushes since there's a whole area of it missing, or apply evenly to your face. You're better off simply replacing it.

Is this product ripe for a bacteria bloom?

Bottom line, your makeup won't last forever, but it doesn't need to be replaced as often as many brands would lead you to believe. Obviously, it's smart business for them to tell you that you need to buy new makeup several times a year, but some of it can actually last you for considerably longer. Here are my guidelines:

JUST STOP leaving caps off your makeup products, especially if you store them in a humid environment like your bathroom. They need to be kept closed so that they aren't exposed to too much humidity, which can encourage bacteria growth.

Sponges and powder puffs—wash 'em or toss 'em every single week.

Sponges and powder puffs are some of the grossest items I see in women's makeup kits. Aside from the fact that a dirty sponge or puff is visually unappealing, they can hold on to all sorts of bacteria from your skin, and then you're just patting it right back on every time you apply more makeup. I throw my cotton/fabric puffs into the wash in a lingerie bag every week, and wash my reuseable sponges like a beautyblender with a little Woolite or liquid soap every couple of days. Disposable sponges are easy to purchase in drugstores and are good for one to two uses each. If your foundation came with a sponge, you should wash it or replace it with a different sponge once it's too dirty or broken down.

Mascara, liquid liner—three to four months.

These are the products that actually do need to be replaced often. Not only does oxygen gets trapped into their tubes, drying out the formula, but heaven forbid you have any eye issues like conjunctivitis or blepharitis because the minute you put the applicator back in the tube, it contaminates everything. You just don't want to mess around when it comes to your eye health.

Tweezers—three to twelve months.

Not everyone has tweezers, but if you are a plucker, when the edge of your tweezers gets dull, it can't grip firmly onto your brow hair. Not only does that make it super frustrating, but it can also be painful to pull out that little hair. Even worse, it can break the follicle, which can lead to ingrown hairs. How often your tweezers need to be sharpened or replaced depends on how often you use them. Companies like Tweezerman offer free sharpening if you mail them in.

JUST STOP thinking that all tweezers are created equal. In order to get the best grip and pull on tiny little brow hairs, they need to be made of high-quality, surgical-grade steel that is extremely thin and sharp on the edge. Thicker-edged tweezers are going to make your work all the more difficult and frustrating because they simply cannot grip the hairs as well. Spend the twenty dollars on high-quality ones.

Cream eye shadow, gel eyeliner—six to twelve months.
Creams and gels can dry out pretty quickly, which you'll see when they start to crack or shrink away from the sides of the container. To keep them pliable for longer, make sure to replace the lid right away, or turn the jar upside down on a flat surface while it's open and not in use. Here's a great little trick—to salvage them when they are dry, add a few eye drops and stir with a toothpick. It softens them right up. The most important thing with these products is to keep your makeup brushes clean and sanitized so that you they don't transmit germs back and forth into your eyes or your skin.

Eye, lip, and brow pencils—one year.
The tip of an eye pencil can get a white crust on it, but don't worry—that's just a little dried saline. With all pencils—brow, eye, lip—sharpen the tip and give a spritz with rubbing alcohol, and you're good to go. After about a year, though, the waxy pencil can start to shrink away from the holder, harden, and then tug on your lid or lips when you apply, which

means it's dried out and needs to be replaced. Obviously, if you have a cold sore or an eye infection, either sanitize your pencil with every single use, or better yet, toss it and start fresh.

Eyelash curler—one year.

Not everyone uses a lash curler, but if you do, you must be sure to wipe the little bumper pad clean after every use and swap in a replacement pad every six months. If you don't replace the little pad, you run the risk of building up so much product on it that it can stick to your lashes and pull them out, or worse, if the pad gets very worn down, it can snap your lashes right off. It's a huge makeup tragedy when your lashes snap off, so believe me, taking care of your lash curler is worth the few seconds of attention.

Foundation and concealer—twelve to eighteen months.

The easiest ways to keep your foundation and concealer fresh is to avoid putting your fingers into them and/or not to unscrew the container if it is airtight. Once fingers/air/light/moisture are allowed in, colors can oxidize, consistencies can thicken, and bacteria can grow. If you don't use your foundation regularly and don't really know how old it is, follow your nose. If it smells slightly sour, it's a surefire indication that it's past its prime.

Lipstick and lip gloss—one to two years.

When exposed to air, many lip glosses can thicken and become uncomfortable to wear. Lipsticks can easily be sprayed or wiped with rubbing alcohol to kill germs, and because they are both emollient formulas, most don't dry out easily.

Cream blush—one to three years.

Most cream blushes have plenty of emollients in them, which means that they won't break down or change color easily. You may see some condensation on them, which can easily be blotted away. As long as you keep unwashed fingers out of them or always use a clean makeup brush, the risk of bacterial growth is low.

Powder for face and cheeks, eye shadow—two to three years.
Most powders have a pretty long shelf life. The problems come when you cross-pollinate, meaning, when the oils from your skin, makeup, or skincare products mix with your powders, transferred there from your makeup brushes. If you see small, shiny speckles or splotches develop on the surface of your powders, blushes, or bronzers, that's a coating of oil left behind from your other products, creating a film on the surface. You can try to lightly scrape the film away with a small butter knife, but if the oils have sunk in too deep, it's a lost cause because your brush just won't be able to pick up product anymore. Also, some powders can oxidize and change color over time. As long as you are okay with that, then there's no reason to rush right out to buy something new.

Makeup brushes—indefinite.
If you care for your brushes and keep them clean, a good-quality makeup brush can last for years and years. Makeup brushes need to be replaced when they shed too much, feel rough on the skin, have lost their shape or have dented/broken/misshapen bristles. If the bristles don't look and feel smooth, they aren't going to give a smooth application.

HOW TO WASH YOUR MAKEUP BRUSHES

You can buy a specific brush cleanser or soap, but any gentle detergent will work fine, such as Woolite or Dreft. Dish detergent will work for synthetic fiber brushes but will dry out natural hair ones.

- Fill a mug one-third full with warm water taking care not to fill it above the point at which the brush handle meets the metal base of the bristles, aka the ferrule.
- Add about a quarter-size drop of detergent.
- Swirl the brushes in the water. For synthetic or very stained brushes, you can then also gently swirl on a plastic cleansing mat or glove (such as the one from Sigma) or in the palm of your hand.
- Holding the tip of the brush down, rinse under warm, running water, gently moving the bristles back and forth until the soap bubbles are gone.
- Gently squeeze excess water from the brush head in a paper towel or dish towel.
- Reshape the brush head, and place flat on a counter with the bristles hanging over the edge. This will allow 360-degree air circulation for faster drying, ensure that water won't drip into the handle to loosen it, and preserve the shape of the bristles.

Just so we're clear—the number one reason to get rid of your makeup is if it has become contaminated in some way. Let me just reiterate what every adult in the world should already know: DO NOT SHARE MAKEUP. EVER. WITH ANYONE. It's not nice to transmit your ailments to others, knowingly or unknowingly, and heaven forbid you are exposed to theirs. Germs do nothing to enhance your beauty and let me tell you, as someone who had to wear her glasses to senior prom due to an unsightly and uncomfortable eye infection, it's a risk you do not want to take.

JUST STOP thinking that it's okay to apply makeup from a store display. A sales associate can help you clean and sanitize what you want to try, but you should never touch your fingers or lips to any display makeup. Who knows how many fingers have been in it, and what they were in before. Same goes for makeup brushes. Always ask the sales associate or makeup artist to make sure they are clean and sanitized.

Sticky Spirits

I bet you're thinking—wow. I never realized exactly how many lipsticks I have, and they're almost all the same color. Maybe you're also wondering, why do I have a dozen lip liners when I rarely wear any of them, or four black eyeliner pencils, or two of the same shade of blush? You could be asking yourself why do I have three eye shadow palettes where one color is worn down to the pan and none of the other colors have been touched? What's this empty compact doing here? Seriously, why did I keep this empty compact?

Now is the time to acknowledge the sticky spirits in your beauty collection—the ones that you can't seem to let go of—but also think clearly about what exactly it is you need to keep in your kit.

- **MAKEUP BRUSHES**—Most women have four to six in total, but it's not necessary to have more than ten to twelve at the most. Multipurpose brushes are best, ones you can use with several different products: 1) foundation/blush/highlighter, 2) bronzer/powder, 3) eye shadow, 4) eye crease and detail 5) concealer/blender 6) pencil brush for eyeliner and spot concealing. So now ask yourself—

    Does it feel rough on the skin?

    Does it shed?

    Does it have a uniform shape?

Does it blend with ease?

Do I know what to do with it?

- **PRIMER/EYE PRIMER**—OPTIONAL, but ideally one for face and one for eyes.

  Does it hold your makeup in place all day long?

  Does it prevent you from getting shiny?

  Does it prevent creasing/fading?

- **FOUNDATION**—one for fall/winter and one a shade deeper for spring/summer.

  Does it look good in photographs?

  Does it irritate your skin or make you break out?

  Does it change color (oxidize) on your skin?

  Does it accentuate your pores, dry patches, or fine lines?

  Does it feel comfortable to wear?

  Does the color match your neck and chest?

- **CONCEALER**—one concealer for the undereyes and to cover blemishes on the face. If you have particular issues in either area, such as extreme dryness, discoloration, or cystic acne, a separate concealer to address each area may be preferred.

  Does it cover your discoloration?

  Does it crease?

  Does it make your skin look dry/crepey?

  Does it last all day?

- **POWDER**—just one.

  Does it accentuate your pores?

Does it make your skin look dry?

Does it feel comfortable to wear?

Does it make you look too pale/too dark?

- **BRONZER**—just one.

  Does it make you look orange?

  Does it make you look dirty/muddy?

  Does it apply too dark or too light?

  Is it easy to blend?

- **HIGHLIGHTER/LUMINIZER**—just one.

  Does it make your skin look oily?

  Is it too pink, too gold, or too silver for your complexion?

  Does it accentuate your pores or fine lines?

- **BLUSH**—one in a peachy tone and one in a pinky tone.

  Does it look like a natural flush?

  Does it accentuate your pores or fine lines?

  Is it easy to blend?

  Does it last all day?

- **EYE SHADOW**—three to four—one for your lid, one for your crease, one to two to line or add details.

  Does it crease?

  Does it accentuate fine lines?

  Does it make your skin look dry?

  Does it fade or last all day?

  Does it provide a special effect for a special occasion?

- **EYELINER**—one deep color, one softer color.

  Does it apply smoothly?
  Does it smudge?
  Does it fade?
  Is it difficult to remove?

- **EYE BROW PENCILS/POWDERS, ETC.**—just one.

  It is easy to apply?
  Does it last all day?

- **MASCARA**—just one, but one that can be layered.

  Does it clump?
  Does it smudge?
  Does it flake?
  Does it make the lashes feel brittle?
  Is it difficult to remove?
  Does it make your eyes water?

- **LIP PENCIL**—OPTIONAL, but if you want one, get a nude tone
  that generally matches your lips.

  Is it much darker or much lighter than your lips?
  Does it match a specific lipstick?
  Does it apply smoothly?
  Does it bleed into the lip lines?

- **LIP GLOSS**—one to two that can be worn alone and one to two that
  can be layered.

  Does it feel sticky, thick, or tacky on your lips?
  Does it dry out your lips?

Does it bleed into the lip lines?

Can it be worn alone or only paired with a lipstick?

Does it have a pleasant fragrance/flavor?

Is it kissable?

• **LIPSTICK**—Everyone has TOO MANY!! And all in the same color family! Whittle it down to three to six in a variety of colors ranging from nude to rose to peach, and three different textures—sheer/balm, satin, creamy/opaque.

Does it wear well?

Does it dry out your lips?

Does it bleed into the lip lines?

Can it be worn alone or only paired with a lip gloss?

• **OTHER TOOLS** like eyelash curlers, tweezers, sponges, etc. —ALL OPTIONAL.

If you pluck your brows, one pair of tweezers.

If you curl your lashes, one lash curler.

If you use a makeup sponge, one reusable sponge, such as a beautyblender or a pack of disposable sponges such as Studio 35.

Pencil sharpener if necessary.

Magnifying mirror if necessary.

Two powder puffs, if necessary. One should always be clean.

Now, at this point, while you have started to say good-bye to the Ghost of Beauty Past, you have not yet had the pleasure of meeting the Ghost of Beauty Yet to Come, so you may be wondering whether you are the best judge of what to keep and what to toss. I promise you, you are—and if you're still not convinced, I promise you that I am. You know instinctively what you like and what you don't. What I'll show you as we move through this book is how to select more friendly ghosts, WHAT TO DO with them, and HOW TO DO it. As we move through the Lazy Perfection method, you'll start to learn about color, texture, and finish, and pick up technical tips and the tricks you need to apply a simple and lovely makeup routine that works for you. By the time we're done, you'll have all the skills you need to be Lazy Perfection personified, a veritable TPW, and Lazy Perfection will come as naturally to you as wine to a book club.

Friendly Ghosts

Congratulations. You've arrived at the last step in the Lazy Perfection Purge routine. I want you to take all your makeup—everything left after the purge. Put it in a basket, box, or bag—and leave it in your closet or another part of your home.

Do not put it back into your bathroom. Do not put it back on your vanity. Do not return it to wherever it lives.

The reason to do this is the last part of the Lazy Perfection Purge, and the MOST IMPORTANT part. This is when you will find out what you really and truly NEED and LOVE in your makeup kit.

Over the course of the next month, you should only pull from this basket or box what you need to use, when you need to use it. Everything else should be left untouched. In a month, it's likely you will have applied makeup for a number of situations—work, weekends, lunches, dinners, dates, parties, carpool, the gym, soccer games . . .

So now you can take the very last step on the Lazy Perfection Purge journey and—GET RID OF ANYTHING YOU HAVE NOT TOUCHED IN THE LAST MONTH. What you will be left with are your Lazy Perfection Essentials, the friendly ghosts who live in your makeup bag.

Ghost of a Chance

Once you have your Lazy Perfection Essentials set aside, they need to be organized in a way that keeps them all visible, giving you more of an opportunity to use and enjoy them more. Arrange them in a drawer liner, a box, or a container, lined up or lain out flat, as long as you get your eyes on each and every item. Cosmetics bags are small and convenient, but you can't see all your makeup when it's stacked on top of each other and jumbled together. And the stuff that's out of sight/out of mind . . . well, if you don't miss that in a couple of weeks as well, you should probably go ahead and purge that, too.

Voilà. Now you can begin to enjoy the Ghost of Beauty Present and get prepared for the Ghost of Beauty Yet to Come.

CHAPTER TWO

A Mantra for Makeup

IN THIS AGE OF CELEBRITY OBSESSION AND SOCIAL MEDIA influencers, makeup hardly seems like a spiritual pursuit. In fact—it can feel like just the opposite, where instead of looking inward for peace and tranquility, we look to the perfectly arched eyebrow as the height of personal fulfillment (although achieving it *can* require the dedication and focus of a monk). Maybe there's a chorus of Instagram yogis who chant a mantra of LIP LINER-LASHES-HIGHLIGHTER-CONTOUR and maybe it works.

While makeup is, on the surface, well, on the surface, I believe there is also a spiritual side to it, the side that elevates us from being mere mortals to being better, happier mortals. Fine, that's not spirituality in the truest sense, but being happy about how we look is the primary objective of Lazy Perfection.

It's the power of positivity, like the Secret. If you feel good about yourself, you put out positive energy, and then that energy gets reflected back at you, which is clearly another reason why TPW is so appealing—it actually feels good to be around her because her vibe is so nice. I don't think it's possible to overstate how impactful the relief that comes with covering up a blemish can be, or even getting a smooth application of eyeliner. When we feel good about ourselves, we interact differently with the world around us.

Just like any other therapeutic practice, my Lazy Perfection methodology requires some goal setting and a willingness to look clearly at your objectives. In this chapter, I am going to guide you through a series of scenarios with the hope that you will relate to one or more of them, recognize your emotional connection with makeup and beauty, and then set yourself on a path to a fresh, simple, and satisfying beauty routine with your Beauty Intention in mind. To be clear, this is not Psychology 101, and it's not a vision quest. But a little introspection and perspective will lead you to a more gratifying relationship with your appearance—and your confidence will soar. Chanting is not required in the Lazy Perfection method, but I am going to ask you to reach deep to try to identify your Beauty Intention and come up with your own Makeup Mantra.

Beauty Enlightenment

One of the first things I do when I meet with a private client is ask her what she hopes to get out of her makeup session with me. This throws a lot of women for a loop, because the answer seems so obvious—I want to look good. But there's more to your Beauty Intention than that.

If you are seeking out Lazy Perfection, I imagine you are not a professional makeup artist. In fact, my guess is that you feel pretty uncertain about your artistry skills, and you probably are unsure about how good your makeup looks. And like so many of the women I work with, you can't put your finger on exactly what's "off" about it.

That's okay. Lazy Perfection isn't for professional makeup artists. I don't expect you to come in with all the answers or to be able to self-assess. One of the first steps on the path to Lazy Perfection is about knowing why you're on it, and I'm here to help you get to the core of your spiritual relationship with your superficial face.

Rhymes with Hunger . . .

I work with lots and lots of women, and in my experience, the number one, top-of-the-heap, alpha reason they come to see me is—*They want to look YOUNGER.* Legions of women out there wake up one day, with a life that's generally joyful and fulfilling, and then they look in the mirror only to find their mother reflected back at them. Even worse, it's their "now" mother, not the one in the photo from twenty-five years ago. Yikes.

So what does looking "younger" mean to you? Like so many women these days, we are caught up in the idea that youth is beautiful, and having worked on models as young as twelve years old, I have to agree. Smooth, unblemished skin, not yet showing signs of sun damage, broken capillaries, the ravages of gravity, or the exhaustion that comes with all the stresses of adulthood—well, it's just lovely.

Remember being able to stay awake until all hours and still get up early the next day feeling fresh, energetic, and looking great? Remember wondering why anyone would bother using concealer? Remember never wearing blush because your cheeks were always rosy?

We all know we can't turn back the clock. There's no way our skin will ever look the way it did when our hormones were firing up for the first time (which, lest we forget, came with its own set of issues) or before we knew that long days at the beach would leave freckles and fine lines percolating under the surface.

It's impossible to look the way we did when we were young, but there are lots of ways to look "younger"—like we have a fresh, healthy glow, are well rested, and are putting out a confident, beautiful vibe.

Time Travel

In all honesty, I am conflicted about the whole "anti-aging" angle on beauty. On the one hand, yes—I miss my old neck and would love to say hello to my smooth eyelids again. They were beloved friends that I took for granted.

On the other hand, I hate that I and so many other women have been made to feel ashamed by the fact that we are getting older and that nature's course isn't good enough. Society's impossible standard of beauty is sometimes demoralizing. We are bombarded with images of women (and men) who are able to avail themselves of all the latest and greatest skincare products and services, not to mention amazing lighting and the magic of retouching. Aging "gracefully" may not actually exist. Unless you are Sharon Stone, in which case you are the hottest damn member of AARP ever.

But there's a third hand here. I and many women in their thirties, forties, and beyond haven't been able to wholeheartedly embrace aging gracefully because we're simply not ready to lose the sense of power and confidence that comes from looking our best, and since we associate aging with a decline in our physical beauty, looking our best is easily referred to as looking "younger."

A few years ago, I was perfectly fine tossing the "anti-aging" phrase around, allowing myself to get caught up in the idea that I could somehow find a way to look and feel the way I did when I was young. But I am willing to bet that if you don't know how old I am, you'll have a hard time guessing. That's because instead of worrying about looking younger, I am focused on making the most of how I look now, in real time, by embracing Lazy Perfection. Liking how you look and using the right makeup and makeup techniques will ensure you don't become a time traveler and so can just hold in place, looking great.

Feeling All the Feelings

So, we've established that you want to look fresher and you want to look more youthful, but now let's pin down your objective a little more clearly. How do you FEEL about your beauty routine? What has led you to the pursuit of Lazy Perfection?

I never learned how to apply makeup, and now it's time.

I hear from women ALL THE TIME that no one ever taught them how to apply makeup or that their mom never wore makeup, and so they never had a role model.

If you talk to women whose mothers did wear makeup, we all have a common memory of sitting in her room, the smell of her perfume in the air, watching her get all dolled-up for a night out. My clearest memory of my mother's beauty routine was of a cream blush shaped like a lollipop that she would swirl onto each cheek and then blend with her fingers. She was gorgeous, glamorous, ethereal, and I wanted to be just like her.

But there are plenty of moms who just weren't into makeup. Plenty of them still aren't, and that's okay, too.

I have never worn makeup but now I feel like I could benefit from it.

Yup. It sucks. As time marches on, our faces march along with it. Skin thins, discoloration and flaws become more visible, and gravity lures our fatty tissue, eyelids, jawlines, and necks down to its deplorable depths. And to add insult to injury, our cell renewal slows, so what once regenerated seemingly overnight now moves at a glacial pace.

Fear not. Lazy Perfection is first and foremost a way to revitalize your appearance in a natural, fresh way. Your complexion will glow again. Your eyes will "pop" once more, and you'll have a bounce in your beauty step again.

I have been using the same makeup since high school.

No matter how you slice it, teenagers wear their makeup differently than adults, even if they wear very little. When you are a teenager, you can get away with a lot more than you can as an adult. Your math teacher may not have balked at your electric blue eyeliner, but your employer might. I know it's not fair that we are judged for our appearances, even though we may be eminently qualified for our jobs, but in many offices, that's still just the way it is. That's not to say that we shouldn't still have fun with makeup and experiment a bit, but now we need to be aware of doing it in an appropriate way. I tell my teen clients (and my teen daughters) all the time that it's human nature to judge, so wouldn't you rather be judged for who you are than what you look like? Our makeup needs to grow up with us.

I want to be taken seriously at my job.

Makeup can be a distraction, whether you're wearing too much or not enough. It's that annoying human nature thing again—we judge each other based on appearance. I have clients who struggle with dark circles and are tired of their coworkers asking them if they're feeling okay. I have worked with women who are in a male-dominated industry and want to feel more powerful and confident when going toe-to-toe with their counterparts. And I have worked with women who have a crippling fear of public speaking and are too nervous to stand up and be scrutinized.

I'm sorry if this isn't a politically correct thing to say, but in many offices, if you fall at one end or the other of the beauty spectrum—looking either underdone or overdone—you are going to be harshly judged. If history has taught us anything, it's that women are still frustratingly held to a higher standard when it comes to our appearance.

I want to look good in photographs.

I think we can all agree that in this digital age, it's disheartening to be tagged in a photo where we look less than our best. The idea that an ex-boyfriend might see a photo where our double chin has tripled or our undereyes look subterranean strikes fear into the hearts of women everywhere.

You might be rolling your eyes and thinking that I'm being ridiculous, but our pictures are out there everywhere these days. On social media. In our LinkedIn profiles. On dating apps. Even when a prospective employer googles us . . . So let's not kid ourselves. Looking good in a photo is actually *important*.

If you're wearing old-fashioned makeup, or the texture of your foundation is making your skin look dry, it will show up in your picture. Believe me, spending a few minutes on your makeup application can make all the difference in the world to how your image presents on the screen of someone's iPhone. Lazy Perfection is a selfie-savior.

JUST STOP posing for photos with a cocker spaniel side-tip of your head. Here is how to pose, the Lazy Perfection way—

- Jut your chin out slightly and tip it up a teensy bit. This makes your neck look longer and takes out some of the shadow under your chin.
- Flatten your tongue into the roof of your mouth. This makes a turkey neck look trimmer and less fowl.
- Raise your eyebrows (or just do the best you can, my fellow Botoxians) and then relax your eyes. This will make them look less squinty.
- Keep your head straight to the camera but turn your shoulders and hips slightly away. This will make your whole body look slimmer.
- And if the photographer is aiming the camera up at you, yell at him to STOP IMMEDIATELY! The most flattering angle is when the camera is raised up higher than eyeline and is pointing down.

I don't want to look tired.

Sleep deprivation is a very hot topic these days, with studies showing over and over again how getting good sleep can boost our intellectual abilities, our interpersonal skills, and our health and fitness levels. But let's focus on the more superficial. Being exhausted can make our complexions look dull or sallow, cause inflammation and dark circles, or even incite the ugly wrath of acne.

The good news is that Lazy Perfection can help you fake being bright-eyed and fresh-faced, even if you don't feel particularly like it.

I like makeup, but I have no idea what I'm doing.

It always surprises me when women who love makeup and who do a nice job of putting it on feel as though they are flying by the seat of their pants. Lazy Perfection doesn't prescribe a strident list of DOs and DON'Ts—if there's makeup you love and enjoy wearing, far be it from me to take that away from you. What I'll show you is how you can make small adjustments in both color and technique that will elevate and polish your look.

I am newly single, and I would like to meet someone.

Updating your makeup is way less permanent than getting a haircut, so if you're looking for a reset and an easy way to reclaim your sexy, this is the method for you. Going through a breakup is hard enough without having to feel like you're not pretty enough or young enough. Lazy Perfection will show you how to reengage with your beauty routine and get your mojo going again. Remember, when you put out the energy that you feel gorgeous, that energy will come back to you. And all it takes is a little bit of effort with your makeup.

I need a routine that's fast but effective.

I feel you. Some days I have less than five minutes to get ready before I am late for school drop-off, and other days, I have to do my makeup in the car. Lazy Perfection fully accounts for the crazy lives we all lead, and if putting on your makeup on the train is your standard-case-scenario, then you will love the tips and tricks for getting a simple, flattering, imprecise look that makes you look refreshed, but can be done on the run.

Makeup overwhelms me.

Yup, there's a lot of it out there, and it can be difficult to narrow down your choices to just the few items that will work for you. My Lazy Perfection method isn't only for choosing the makeup you want to wear, but also for how to go shopping for it, and how to put it on. Lazy Perfection is like a deep, cleansing breath. It'll help you relax into the process and enjoy it more.

Realistic Rouge

So now that you've identified the reasons you are seeking Beauty Enlightenment, there's one last thing to consider—reality. This is the reality of what you are willing to put into Lazy Perfection and how lazy or perfect you really want to be. There's no right or wrong answer—just what's right or wrong for you.

- How much time are you willing to put into your makeup routine? Five minutes? Thirty minutes? Your beauty objective cannot be achieved unless it's in line with the amount of time you are willing to spend. The more detailed and technical your application routine, the longer it will take to complete. Every Lazy Perfection step is designed to work efficiently and together in harmony, but it's up to you to decide how many steps you want to take.

- Do you have the technical skills or are you willing to learn them?

One of the most common refrains I hear from my clients is that when they don't feel successful with a particular step in their makeup application, they simply give up. So ask yourself whether, realistically, you have the skills you need to get a clean cat-eye swoop or a contoured cheek, and if not, are you willing to take the time to learn?

JUST STOP beating yourself up about not being able to apply your makeup like a pro. It's not something that comes naturally to most people and, as with everything in life, practice makes perfect. I recommend test driving new makeup techniques at bedtime to get a feel for them. That way, you can simply wash it off if you make a mistake instead of having to either start from scratch or face the rest of your day feeling self-conscious.

- Know yourself and your limitations. Are you someone who is always running late? Do you care whether your mascara looks fluffy or spiky? Can you be bothered to deal with a ten-step beauty routine? It's the "You can't have it both ways" conundrum. Acknowledging whether you're simply not able to focus on a lengthy makeup routine will help you determine which Lazy Perfection steps are the right ones for you.

Purposefully Pretty

It's time to look with purpose at where all this introspection has led you. Think of this step as your Beauty Third Eye, the one that shows you your truest path to Lazy Perfection.

There are three Lazy Perfection Beauty Tracks:

Simple

The Simple Path is just that—a pared-down, fast, übernatural plan for making small but impactful changes to your makeup application. It's just a couple of steps above being barefaced, but will give you prettier skin, clearer eyes, and a fresher, more modern look. If you need to be ready fast, this is for you. If you have young kids tugging at you, you're athletic and outdoorsy, lead a casual lifestyle, have a very minimalistic personal style and don't want to be bothered with tricky techniques, this is the track for you. It's not fussy or complicated—only flattering. If your beauty ideals are Shailene Woodley, Gigi Hadid, Gisele Bündchen, Jessica Biel, Gwyneth Paltrow, Ellen Pompeo, Jamie Lee Curtis, Padma Lakshmi, or Helen Mirren then you will be at home on the Lazy Perfection Simple Track.

Sophisticated

The Sophisticated Track builds on what the Simple Path introduced and is where most Lazy Perfectionites live. It's a look that is put together without being overdone, where your features are set off to their best effect without your makeup looking obvious, or even visible at all. To achieve it, you'll add in a few more products to your routine and learn a couple of new tricks, but will continue to employ small but significant steps that refine and enhance your look. If you work in a professional environment, have meetings to attend, are involved with volunteer or professional organizations, like to get dressed up for lunches or dinners out, are dating, or simply want to step up your beauty look, this is the Lazy Perfection Track for you. If your beauty ideals are Jennifer Aniston, Emma Watson, Blake Lively, Eva Mendes, Julia Roberts, Nicole Kidman, Anna Kendrick, Lucy Liu, Demi Moore, Beyoncé, Halle Berry, or Sandra Bullock then you will feel right at home on the Sophisticated Track.

Sexy

The Sexy Lazy Perfection Track builds on both the Simple and Sophisticated ones, adding in a few more details to the look to give an added level of glamour. Your eyes will sparkle, your complexion will glow, your cheeks will look sculpted and radiant, and your lips will look plump and, oh yes, sexy.

This is for evenings out, parties, galas, when you know you'll have your photo taken and splashed all over social media, a hot date, or for times when you want to infuse your look with added drama. Never overworked, never overdone, even the Lazy Perfection Sexy Look is about natural beauty and enhancing your features, not trying to change them.

If your beauty ideals are Jennifer Hudson, Sofía Vergara, Megan Fox, Olivia Wilde, Michelle Obama, Penélope Cruz, Angelina Jolie, Sophia Loren, Emily Ratajkowski, Kerry Washington, Kaley Cuoco, or Catherine Zeta-Jones then you will get so much out of the Lazy Perfection Sexy Track.

Your Makeup Mantra

No matter what track you choose, always remember that Lazy Perfection is about looking natural and beautiful, and making the most of your features.

Now, sit down, take a deep breath in, and repeat this chant after me . . . I AM LAZY PERFECTION (*ding*).

CHAPTER THREE

Girl Scout Guide

BUST OUT YOUR KHAKI VESTS AND GET READY TO SEW ON SOME
patches, ladies, because we're going to take a little excursion, Girl Scout
style. Now that you've purged your bathroom of all the clutter and noise
and you've set your Beauty Intention, the last step in getting ready for
your new Lazy Perfection beauty routine is knowing how to always be
prepared—like a Girl Scout, only without the cookies, and you're going
shopping for makeup instead of camping. If you ask me, navigating the
beauty counters in a department store is every bit as daunting as living in
the woods for a week, but don't worry. I'm here to be your Scout Master.

Always Be Prepared

I know that I am asking you to put some effort into your beauty routine before you even get your makeup on, and I don't want you to actually go shopping until you read the rest of the information I provide in the chapters coming up, but these are the things that you need to think about in order to streamline. Remember, Lazy Perfection isn't lazy in the sense that you can do nothing. It's lazy in the sense that once you get prepared for your updated, fresh look, you'll be able to do way less, way better. Less stress, less anxiety, more satisfaction—a satisfaction greater than any Thin Mint could ever bring you (unless you have PMS, in which case the Thin Mints win every time). So, let's put on our backpacks (fine, purses), and head out to buy some makeup. But first, there are a few things you should know.

Into the Woods

Shopping for makeup is a tricky business. Even as a makeup artist and a beauty expert, I find navigating a makeup department akin to weed-whacking my way through a forest. It's sensory overload. There are dangers lurking everywhere, so I need to keep moving, and the minute I stop, something unseen scuttles through the underbush that puts me very much on edge. Yeah—it's not really that dramatic, but you get what I mean. It's a challenging environment.

I find that one of two things happens to me when I get to the makeup counter—I'm either completely mistrustful and suspicious of what the salesperson has to say because I know it is her job to sell me things or I overspend on too many products that I won't use more than a couple of times because I am just so gosh darned susceptible to suggestion. Yes, even me, a makeup artist. If someone at a store swears that a new lipstick color is going to rock my world and make me feel like I have been directly touched by the hands of the gods, then I am all in! The only problem is, and I'm sure you can relate, I get that new lipstick home and try it on in the safety of my own room, with my own familiar lighting, and guess what . . . it ends up in my makeup drawer, creating clutter and adding to my already sizable guilt at having spent my hard-earned dollars on something I won't use.

But there are lots of things you can do to avoid these scenarios. Armed with a little information about how to navigate your shopping experience and what your actual beauty needs are, you can and will come away feeling like the whole experience was Lazy Perfection. Seamless, simple, and satisfying.

Survival of the Fittest

There are millions of reasons women like to go shopping, from the deeply emotional to the spontaneous. No matter what has brought you out of the comfort of your home or through the screen of your computer, the objective is always the same—to bring home something that makes you feel great.

And the salespeople know that. All too well. Which is why shopping for makeup is a bit of a Darwinian experience, where only those who are Beauty-Evolved make it out with products that are just right for them.

Forest Green

Beauty is a MULTIBILLION-dollar industry and one that plays on our emotions and our sense of self. Now, I really don't have any issue with the Beauty-as-a-Business approach. I totally get that it's a machine and that everyone from the counter manager to the pigment formulator, to the shipping assistant at the factory, to the ad executive at the magazine is impacted by what we, the consumers, purchase. And we consumers aren't just paying for the products we buy, but we're also paying for the cost of the packaging, marketing, advertising, celebrity spokespeople, sales-force training, and more. It's all built into the cost of that pretty little product, and believe me, it's a whole lot of green. Big cash.

But shopping for makeup isn't all fun and games. It can be stressful and overwhelming, expensive, and, if not done well, wasteful. So let's take a look at how we can enjoy the experience more, find a way to select products that add value to our kits, and help us to look lovely and come away feeling good about the purchases we make.

JUST STOP thinking that if you see something get a good review on a blog, it's unquestionably a good product. The best and most reputable bloggers will give you their genuine opinions, for better or for worse, which gives their reviews credence but still doesn't guarantee that the product will be suitable for you. There are other bloggers who will give glowing reviews no matter what, which naturally makes them less trustworthy. Often, the brands supply free product, the blogger posts a lovely product review, and so the brand supplies more product. It's a great setup for the bloggers because Yay! Free makeup! and Yay! Something new to post! And since having a steady stream of new content is crucial for bloggers, if their relationship with a brand sours, that content stream dries up. If you are someone who likes to research before you shop, user reviews may give you a more objective sense of the product simply because the reviewers have paid for their items themselves and aren't beholden to the brands.

Department and Specialty Beauty Stores

Let me pause here and just address specialty store and department store makeup artists directly. I know you are likely a good person with good intentions. I know that you probably have some artistry experience. I know you have a hard and competitive job to do. And I know that there is pressure on you to make a sale. Respect to the department store beauty girls all day long. And even more to the perfume ladies who get shot down and shut out all day long. That's got to be demoralizing.

But . . . beauty is still a consumer-focused business, and at the end of the day, if consumers aren't making purchases, there's a ripple effect throughout the industry, so the pressure on salespeople is enormous.

Did you know that at many counters, if you don't make a certain number of sales weekly, you get fired? The job is about MAKING SALES, ladies, but because we the consumer are so emotional about our appearances and so filled with hope about how makeup might transform us, we can sometimes end up making unwise purchases. Because we are emotionally charged when it comes to our appearance, we are susceptible to the pressures the salespeople are under—they can influence our purchases by telling us how great we look, which new color is hot for the season, or how new technology is going to do amazing things for us.

Here are a few tips and tricks for navigating a beauty store so that you'll end up taking home only the products that you will use and love. And not come away with hundreds of dollars of products that will just sit in your drawer.

Around the Campfire

As you walk through the store, salespeople are trained to engage you so that they can continue the conversation and get you on a path to a transaction. They'll draw you in by saying, "Is it still snowing/raining/ gorgeous out there?" or "I love your jacket/purse/shoes . . ." or even a simple "Are you finding everything okay?" As soon as you respond, they have you on the line because you have engaged. Maybe their questions are genuine and their compliments heartfelt, so how do you know whether you can trust them to help you select your beauty products? How can you decide if you want to share your beauty campfire with them?

JUST STOP thinking that you can't switch from one sales associate to another. I know we all want to be polite and not hurt anyone's feelings, but we also want to make smart purchases. If you don't like the first person who approaches you, or the second, you can keep talking to new people until you find the one. Any associate who gets snippy or rude if you move along to someone else isn't someone you'd want to work with anyway, and it's certainly not someone the brands/ stores would be keen on representing them.

Even if you are just browsing or you don't have a particular product you are seeking out, the first step in deciding if someone could be your bestie at the campfire is to decide whether you share a similar beauty aesthetic.

Now, that doesn't mean you should judge them based on their own makeup. Yes, we've already talked about how it's human nature to judge, but store sales associates are often required by their employer to use particular products, apply a certain number of products, or project a designated overall look so that when the customer asks about it, they can answer by pointing to their own faces. You might see a neon pink blush and say, "Wow! This blush is crazy bright" and they can then legitimately respond, "It's not really. I'm wearing it myself today." So their makeup isn't always an accurate reflection of their personal taste. You'll have to dig deeper if you want to get at what it really is.

Sharing Your S'mores

The easiest way to find out if a makeup salesperson's aesthetic is similar to yours is to ask her about it, plain and simple. Maybe you like marshmallows and she doesn't. You need to know that if she is offering to share her s'mores, you like the way she makes them. Here's how you can figure it out:

Can you see her foundation sitting on top of her skin? Does it look like something you would consider to be "natural"? Ask her to describe that foundation, what she likes about it, why she chose it, and whether or not she would recommend it. All you have to say is "What foundation are you wearing?" and then once you have her answer, repeat with questions about her eye shadow, blush, or whatever you're curious about. Her answers will be very revealing.

A good salesperson will ask you questions right back, trying to get the insights that will help her get to the core of the makeup you would like. If she describes her makeup as simple, ask yourself if it seems simple to you. If she describes it as natural, same thing—does it look clean and fresh to you?

Another surefire way to get a read on her aesthetic is to ask for her opinion about a celebrity you admire. Grab a couple of screenshots and keep them on your phone so you can pull them out when you're chatting. You can ask leading questions like "What do you think of this look?" or "What are the steps I need to take to get it?" or "Are there other celebs whose makeup you like more?" Listen to the steps she talks you through and the people she brings up. If you want to rock some Blake Lively but she adores Rihanna, it seems likely that her s'mores aren't going to be cooked the way you like them.

JUST STOP letting a makeup artist get you in her chair before you assess whether you think she's part of your beauty scout troop. She's going to ask you within moments of initiating a conversation whether you want her to do your makeup, because she knows that as soon as she's put any makeup on your face, it's hard, if not impossible, for you to get away without making a purchase. Make her buy you a drink before you commit to dinner, if you know what I mean. Consider it a beauty courtship.

Reading a Beauty Map

So, what if you don't know how to get to the core of your beauty aesthetic? What if you just have a vague sense of what you think is pretty but don't know how to point your compass to it? You need a beauty map, something you can steer by when you're trying to find your way. Consider the beauty brands your landmarks. If you know generally where they are, you're less likely to get lost. All brands fall into five basic categories:

Natural (Bobbi Brown, Laura Mercier, Trish McEvoy, IT Cosmetics, Cover Girl, bareMinerals, Maybelline, Sonia Kashuk, Almay) This look is subtle, simple, and understated with an emphasis on enhancing natural skin tones and textures.

Natural Plus (like Lancôme, Becca, Anastasia, Benefit, Stila, Too Faced, Kevyn Aucoin, Rimmel, e.l.f.) Natural Plus takes a little more effort and a few more products but the end result is still a look that doesn't scream "I am wearing makeup." It has slightly more oomph than natural, but you have to look more closely to see the details.

Glamorous (like Dior, YSL, Charlotte Tilbury, Tom Ford, Armani, Chanel, Gucci, Dolce & Gabbana, Clé de Peau Beauté) More luxury, more drama, more effort. Think Red Carpet. It doesn't have to be heavy-handed, but glamorous makeup looks like makeup, not like you woke up that way.

Colorful/Trendy (like MAC, Make Up For Ever, NARS, Kat Von D, Urban Decay, NYX) Bright colors, specific techniques, designed to be noticed. Think MTV Movie Awards or fashion runway shows. Note: Bright, colorful, and trendy makeup is not generally the Lazy Perfection Look, although elements of it can be incorporated if you're feeling sassy.

Clean/Green Beauty (like W3LL PEOPLE, Juice Beauty, RMS, Ilia, Jane Iredale, Beautycounter, Honest Beauty) These products are more about their ingredients than their style, but tend to lean toward a more natural, simple look.

Winds of Change

A word about Clean Beauty—it's a massively growing category and is going to become increasingly developed and available in the coming years, even at mainstream stores. Ingredients are generally nontoxic, and may also be organic, vegan, gluten-free, cruelty-free, and eco-friendly. I am embracing Clean Beauty myself, adding it to my kit as I find more and more products that are well formulated and equal in quality and performance to conventional beauty products.

Troop Leaders

Bear in mind that when you work with a makeup artist who is representing a certain brand, he or she has been trained in that line, with those products, and is obligated to sell them.

Many department stores now have Beauty Concierges who are not employed by the brands themselves, or on commission from those brands, but have been trained across multiple lines. They don't have the same sales goal pressures as other sales associates and can, therefore, give you a more objective perspective. Call your favorite stores to see if they have one or more on staff.

Side note—Sales associates at specialty stores such as Sephora and Ulta, and at independent boutiques and chains are generally not on commission and are, therefore, more objective about what they will recommend for you.

Campfire Compatible

If you are all in on getting your makeup done and don't have time to assess the compatibility of your tent mate, please know that before you let yourself get colors swiped up and down your face, it is *im.per.a.tive* that you are able to communicate to the artist EXACTLY how you want him or her to make you look.

Familiarize yourself with the basic looks—natural, natural plus, glamorous, trendy—and bring a photograph with you of a makeup look you find appealing. Seriously. One woman's "natural" is another woman's *RuPaul's Drag Race*, so you can't just rely on language. Visual aids are critical.

In-store makeup application is ripe for disappointment, so the more clearly you convey your needs and wants, the more likely it is you will have a gratifying outcome. And no makeup artist worth her salt should be offended if you ask her to make adjustments to your makeup. I always tell my clients that I have no ego in the work I do—the most important thing is that they walk out into the world feeling great.

JUST STOP thinking that you don't have to tip a store makeup artist, even if there is no charge for the service or no minimum purchase required. As long as it's not against store policy—which you should ask ahead of time—a gratuity is customary and very much appreciated.

Self-Guided Scouting

Now, shopping online for makeup is a whole other kettle of fish, but for now we're just going to focus on drugstores and big box stores You get the Lazy Perfection GOLD Merit Badge if you've had a successful self-guided shopping trip to a drugstore. Something for you to know before you go— at most big box and drugstore chains, purchases may be returned even if they have been opened.

If the first step in a successful shopping expedition to a department or specialty store is finding the right person to help you, the first step in a having a successful trip to a drugstore or big box store is to understand what you are looking at. This arms you with information about the products that are most likely to suit your needs, and will allow you to navigate your options.

There are three different characteristics of makeup that you need to evaluate before making any purchase, whether it's for your face, eyes, or lips.

First of all, what CONSISTENCY is right for you? This is the physical state of the makeup you should choose, the texture. In general, dry skin should stay away from dry textures and oily skin should stay away from oily or very wet textures, but there are several different variations of each texture.

> JUST STOP thinking that there's only one makeup that's right for you. There are so many options and so many variations, you can have a sense of what works for you and then experiment to see if there are others. The guidelines I am giving you are subject to your own satisfaction.

Next, what degree of COVERAGE do you like? Meaning, how much of your natural skin do you want to be visible? Many foundations are "buildable," meaning that you can apply more than one layer in order to get more coverage.

And lastly, what FINISH will flatter your skin? Meaning, how much sheen do you want your skin to have? Matte has no sheen, satin looks like natural skin, radiant contains small reflective particles and dewy looks the most hydrated and moisturized.

JUST STOP thinking that you have to fly blind. There are lots of online resources for getting insights into the various consistencies, coverage, and finishes of a product. Blogs like *Temptalia*, *Musings of a Muse*, *British Beauty Blogger*, *Caroline Hirons*, *Beauty Editor*, and *The Beauty Look Book* give detailed breakdowns of all the features, as well as extensive swatch images, and *MakeupAlley* is an excellent online forum for user reviews. I enjoy all these resources because they give honest, unbiased opinions. Just remember, a blogger isn't necessarily a makeup artist or a Lazy Perfection aficionado, so they won't be able to help you determine whether a product is right for you.

If you're shopping online, yes, it's Lazy Perfection in theory . . . but it's a challenge to choose the best makeup without seeing it in person. If you do shop electronically, I would encourage you to research swatches to make sure you get a good color match.

JUST STOP taking virtual makeup apps seriously—they are often not real-world applicable. New apps are rolling out all the time that have cool technology and allow you to load a photo and experiment with new looks, but the problem is whether you'd be able to replicate the same look at home. Apps are fun to play with, but aren't Lazy Perfection–approved for makeup shopping purposes just yet. If you want to check some out just to play, try L'Oréal Makeup Genius, Mary Kay, and Sephora.

We're going to dive into what makeup will be best for you in the coming chapters, but in the mean time I offer you congratulations, Girl Scout. You've followed your beauty map, met your campfire bestie, and cooked up some pretty mean s'mores. You've earned your Preparedness badge, and now you're ready to face the forest all on your own.

CHAPTER FOUR

Saving Face

I'M GOING TO BREAK EVERY GOOD STORYTELLER'S RULE AND start with the punch line. Ready? If you take care of your skin, your entire beauty routine will be faster, easier, and more gratifying.

One of the reasons I don't read a lot of magazines or blogs, other than not having the time or the patience (and being super lazy), is because every time I do there's another story about a new technique, procedure, or ingredient that's going to be a skincare *savior*, and quite frankly, trying to keep up with it all stresses me out. I always feel like I am falling behind and if I don't jump in and slather it all over my face, I am going to wake up tomorrow looking like the Crypt Keeper.

Face Time

I want you to know super clearly and very early on in this chapter that *Lazy Perfection* doesn't mean that I recommend you do *nothing* to take care of your skin. In fact, this is the part of your beauty routine that probably needs the *most* time and attention because it is the real foundation of your appearance—the physical foundation, not the kind that comes in a bottle. Sure, you can fake pretty skin, but I assure you with 100 percent certainty that taking five minutes when you wake up and five minutes before bed to care for your skin will not only give you a complexion that's more clear and hydrated, but it will also help protect you from the health risks associated with poor skincare. Yep, health risks. Beauty isn't all fun and games.

In Your Face

So, here's the scoop with skincare. It's a massive, gigantic, monster of a business and is growing at an incredible rate every single day. We are bombarded with information about new technologies that promise tighter, firmer, more lifted skin. Bloggers post every day about how they tried this new product or that new ingredient, or post pictures of the products they use in their ten-step routine. There are ads and articles and celebrity endorsements, and even though TPW won't share what exactly it is she does (because TPW is shrouded in mystery, of course), you just know that it's something more than a bar of soap and water.

So, how can we make our skincare routines simpler and easier, with a good return on investment? Botox every four months can really add up, but then again, so can all the makeup we're buying to try to hide our imperfections. You have to know where to invest your money, time, and energy so that you can get the best routine and results possible.

Keeping a Straight Face

I have to admit that my personal Beauty Intention, to look fresher, trips me up when it comes to skincare. I am as susceptible to marketing and messaging as the next girl—the promise of "instant youth," even though it may come at a steep price, is sometimes too alluring to pass up. I have tried it all—Botox, fillers, lasers, radiofrequency facials, ultrasonic facials, peels, microdermabrasion, dermaplaning, lighteners, brighteners, wrinkle-fighters . . . The truth is that some of them will work for you, some of them won't—and it's tricky to figure out where to spend your time and money.

While I have found some treatments to be helpful add-ons, nothing beats the consistency of a good daily routine. The secret to great skin is to build a routine that both corrects and prevents your complexion woes. There are lots of ways to streamline and simplify and still get beautiful results, and I'm going to talk you through how to do it all in typical Lazy Perfection style.

You know your skin type—Dry, Combination, Normal, Oily, or Sensitive—so just make sure you get yourself on the track that's best suited to your needs.

DRY SKIN—Avoid alcohols; use milky creams and lotions

NORMAL SKIN—Free for all! Creams, Gels, Lotions . . . whatever works for you and feels good on your skin

OILY SKIN—Gels that absorb quickly and cleansers that foam will be your BFFs

COMBINATION SKIN—Avoid creams; stick with lotions

SENSITIVE SKIN—Avoid citrus extracts, fragrances, and high percentages of active ingredients

JUST STOP thinking that coffee, tea, juice, or soda is enough to keep you hydrated. Your body needs good old-fashioned H_2O, and plenty of it. Science might not confirm the impact of hydration on the appearance of the skin, but millions of professionals like makeup artists, models, celebrities, and aestheticians know that your skin absolutely looks better when your body is hydrated.

JUST STOP thinking that just because a product is "Natural" or "Botanical" that it won't irritate your skin. You never know how your body is going to react to something found in nature. If you have environmental allergies, it's not unlikely that your skin will be reactive to at least some botanical ingredients.

Face Value

First and foremost, you need to ask yourself what bothers you about your skin. What's the first thing your eye is drawn to when you look in the mirror? The most common grievances are related to:

- Fine lines and wrinkles
- Enlarged pores
- Redness/rosacea
- Sun damage/dark spots
- Discoloration
- Dull tone
- Dry or dehydrated skin
- Sagging or loss of elasticity
- Inflammation or puffiness
- Sensitive, reactive skin
- Oil production, breakouts, or acne

Unfortunately, unless you have won the genetic lottery or have lived sequestered away from daylight, you are likely to have more than one area of concern. So now you have to ask yourself—how much time are you willing to put into correcting them? How much effort? And how much money?

There are three basic Lazy Perfection Skincare Tracks you can follow:

• Simple

• Sophisticated

• Sexy

Simple Skincare Track

STEP 1—FACE AND FOREMOST

The Golden Rule of Skincare, first and foremost, for EVERYONE, is always WASH YOUR FACE BEFORE YOU GO TO BED. Tipsy? Wash anyway. Exhausted? Wash anyway. Lazy? . . . WASH ANYWAY. This is hardly a groundbreaking tip, but it *always* bears repeating. I come across women all the time who tell me that they don't wash their faces before bed, and it stuns and confuses me. And washing your face before bed "most" of the time isn't building the consistency that skin thrives on for recovery and smooth operation.

JUST STOP using Makeup Remover Wipes every night at bedtime. Sure, they are fast and easy, and yes, once in a while they are fine to use, but so many of them are loaded up with sugars (because that's what breaks down your makeup) that they can strip your skin of its good oils and leave a film on the surface through which your other skincare products can't penetrate. Wipes are for eye makeup or Emergency Use Only.

I can't get into bed without washing away the dirt and grime that has accumulated on my skin—no way, no how. It's flat-out gross. And waking up with crusty makeup on my face, smudges around my eyes and pores that are angry at having been treated so carelessly? I just can't do it.

We live in a world suffused with pollution, germs, and dirt . . . by the end of the day, our skin has collected the grit that floats in the air, not to mention the number of things we touch over the course of the day, from food to doorknobs, to mobile phones and computers . . . things that are covered in germs, grease, and grime that get transferred to our faces. I don't mean to alarm you, but in case you aren't already aware, we live in a dirty world.

"But, I don't even wear any makeup," you may be saying to yourself. Well, let me tell you what will happen to your skin if you don't wash away the grime before bed—with or without having added makeup into the mix. Your pores will get clogged with the oils and grime that land on our skin just from walking outside, leading to blackheads, whiteheads, or inflammation. Without daily cleansing that stimulates circulation in the skin and helps with cell renewal and turnover, it'll get dull. And the natural production of the good oils in your skin—the ones that help hydrate and firm, will be disrupted, throwing off the natural rhythm of rejuvenation that happens while we sleep. If you don't wash your face daily, you will be left having to struggle with more foundation, more concealer, and more disappointment as you try to make your skin look pretty.

As for washing in the morning, unless your skin is combination or oily, a rinse with warm water, or a light sweep with a damp cotton round, is probably enough to remove what's left of your skincare products from the night before, and then you are ready to move on. If you're combination, oily, or prone to breakouts, a simple rinse followed by a sweep with some toner may be enough.

STEP 2—WIPE THAT SKIN OFF YOUR FACE

Exfoliation is the purposeful removal of dead skin cells and is the fastest way to get your skin looking fresher. Your skin naturally sheds cells every day, this just helps wipe them away even faster. By speeding up cell turnover you get these benefits:

- Unclogging pores/blackheads
- Reducing the size of your pores
- Improving skin tone and radiance
- Fading pink scars or other superficial marks on the skin

By clearing away the old, you are literally making way for the new—new skincare ingredients that can penetrate deeper and be more effective, and new collagen and cells that will improve tone, brightness, and texture. It usually takes twenty-eight days or more for old skin cells to run through their natural cycle of sloughing, but by helping them along, your skin will look smoother and fresher faster. You don't need to exfoliate every single day, but three to four times per week will have a big impact on your glow.

There are three different forms of exfoliation:

CHEMICAL—Using skincare ingredients that cause a microshedding of dead skin cells, allowing new skin cells to generate faster.

MECHANICAL—Using a device, such as a facial cleansing brush to assist with the sloughing away of dead skin cells.

PHYSICAL/MANUAL—Using your hands to apply a textured "scrub" to rub and roll away dead skin cells, or using a loofah or washcloth.

JUST STOP thinking that manual exfoliation with a scrub is the safest, easiest, and most effective. Nuts, seeds, and sugar particles have rough edges that can make tiny tears in the skin, which over time can lead to microscarring or inflammation. If you must manually exfoliate, look for particles that dissolve, like biodegradable, water-soluble beads, or just use a washcloth.

Truthfully, you don't really even need to know exactly what it is you're treating because exfoliation addresses so many of the most common skincare issues we face. Really. We could call this step *Clueless Perfection*.

There are a couple of amazing multipurpose treatment ingredients in particular. They are the skincare Wonder Twins. Introducing here—the Dynamic Duo—the Saviors of the Skin—the Exfoliating Extravaganza . . . *retinoid* and her charming companion *alpha hydroxy acid*.

These two ingredients are really and truly saviors of the skin. No matter what your skin type, your age, or the issues you want to correct or prevent, they are going to start you on the right path to skin correction by working their multipurpose magic. But do bear in mind that with these ingredients, it's a nighttime path. Lit by the twinkling of fairies and lightning bugs, and sprinkled with dew. Okay, fine, maybe it's not as fanciful as all that, but my point is that you want to be careful about applying retinoids or AHAs during the day as they may make your skin more light-sensitive.

Retin to Sender

Tretinoin (aka Renova or Retin-A) and its over-the-counter cousin Retinol are like Rememberalls (that's a little something for all you Harry Potter nerds out there)—they help you remember what your skin used to look like when you were younger . . . and then make it a reality. There are so many different formulations of tretinoin out there, prescription and nonprescription, in a range of different potencies. Not only do they help speed skin cell turnover, but they also stimulate collagen growth, which leads to smoother texture, improved elasticity, more even coloration, and reduced pore size. It's a skincare Swiss Army Knife.

The caveat, of course, is that the more potent formulations can also be pretty drying or irritating on the skin, and there are lots of people who can't tolerate them—me included. I've always done better with the lesser strength over-the-counter products, but even they can freak my skin out a bit. My advice is to start with an inexpensive, low-dosage Retinol product and see if your skin likes it before stepping it up. Over-the-counter products might take a little longer to show visible results, but for a small investment and less likelihood of irritation, it's worth giving it a try.

An AHA Moment!

Alpha hydroxy acid (aka AHA) sounds a little scary, right? Like something that is used to burn off warts or clean up industrial waste. Not to worry—AHAs are naturally occurring acids that are derived from plants, seeds, leaves, flowers, milks, and fruits. You have probably heard of or tried:

• Glycolic Acid

• Lactic Acid

- Mandelic Acid
- Tartaric Acid

Glycolic is the one most commonly used simply because it's the most researched. It comes in a variety of strengths, ranging from 2 percent up to 70 percent when administered in a dermatologist's office, and can be found in the form of toners, washes, pads, lotions, or creams. As with tretinoin, you can start slowly with a 10 percent over-the-counter product (which is about standard for most retail formulations) and then step it up from there if you want faster results or if it seems that your skin can tolerate a more aggressive percentage. If you want a really aggressive treatment, you can definitely schedule a high percentage peel at a dermatologist's office, but just be prepared for a little downtime during which you'll look about as smooth and flake-free as a snake shedding its skin. It's not pretty, but when you're eventually done shedding, you'll have a baby soft, radiant complexion.

If your skin rejects Retinols, AHAs are the perfect backup plan. And if your skin can tolerate Retinols, lucky you—you can use them in combination with AHAs.

By the way, for all you oily gals out there, AHA has a very cute sibling named BHA (beta hydroxy acid). BHA—most commonly known as salicylic acid—is great for anyone who has acne or breakouts. AHAs can't break down oils, but BHAs can, so when they get into the pores, they dissolve the oils and accumulated dead cells that cause breakouts.

JUST STOP using toners that contain alcohol or are called "astringent." They dry out the surface of your skin without giving you any deep cellular repair. Toners are an optional step, but if you like to use one, look for a water-based formulation that's loaded up with helpful ingredients like antioxidants, AHAs or BHAs that can target specific skin issues, such as oil production, dullness, or uneven texture.

STEP 3—FACE THE MUSIC

This is the fork in the Simple Plan path, where you need to go down a split path. How can you be in two places at the same time? Time-Turner, obviously (too many Harry Potter references?). During the day—protect with SPF. At night—moisturize, moisturize, moisturize. Let's go down the daytime SPF path first.

Facing the Consequences

What I am about to tell you is IMPORTANT stuff.

Remember when I said earlier in this chapter that skincare isn't all fun and games? That it's also about your HEALTH? That's where protection comes in, otherwise you could really have to face the consequences.

You need to wear at least SPF 15 EVERY. SINGLE. DAY. OF THE YEAR. Really, every single one. Rain or shine, indoors or outdoors, makeup or no makeup. Yes, you read that right. Windows protect us from burning, but they won't protect us from damage, so even if you're inside, if you're by a window, you are at risk for sun damage. Getting sun feels great, energizes us, stimulates the production of all sorts of nutrients for energy and growth . . . but it's essentially a sweet, sweet poison.

Some people are able to tolerate the sun better than others, but EVERYONE needs to use a broad-spectrum sunscreen with a minimum SPF of 15 EVERY DAY OF THE YEAR. I know I am repeating myself. It's on purpose.

There are three things you need to understand about SPF:

1) Ultraviolet rays comes in 3 varieties, called broad spectrum, a term you have no doubt heard:
- UVA—A is for Aging. These are the sun rays that cause visible signs of aging like freckles and fine lines, and nonvisible signs of aging that lurk below the surface of our skin, aka sun damage.

- UVB—B is for Burning. These rays vary in strength depending on the time of the year, but are the ones you really want to look out for from a HEALTH standpoint. Yup—these are the cancer-causing rays, and I don't think I need to go on and on about how these should be avoided at all costs
- UVC—These are ultraviolet rays, but because of the ozone layer, they never reach us here on Earth. Yay! Something we don't have to worry about!

2) There are two different types of sunscreen—chemical and physical. **Chemical sunscreens** like avobenzone, oxybenzone, or Mexoryl are the ones that need to be applied thirty minutes before you go out into the sun. They work by absorbing the sun's rays.
Physical Sunscreens (aka mineral sunscreens) like zinc oxide and titanium dioxide, work by blocking and deflecting the sun's rays and are effective immediately.

   The kind you use is entirely up to you and depends on what your skin can tolerate. Chemical sunscreens irritate my skin, whereas my fabulous assistant has an allergy to the oxides. Just use whichever works for you.

3) SPF is the rated level of coverage. It's a complicated rating system and depends on lots of factors, like your skin type, the time of year, and whether or not you're using the correct amount of it, which is between the size of a nickel and a quarter for the face and neck. Basically:
   - SPF 15 blocks 93 percent of the sun's rays
   - SPF 30 blocks 97 percent
   - SPF 50 blocks 98 percent

JUST STOP thinking that a higher SPF gives you significantly more protection. As you can see, the difference from an SPF 15 to an SPF 50 is nominal, so as long as you are using at least SPF 15, you should be covered. Of course, if you have a history of burns, my advice is to start with SPF 50 and then try each of the lower percentages if you wish, to see if there is any difference. Your skin deserves the best care possible and will reward you for your efforts for decades to come!

JUST STOP thinking that a higher SPF means you'll be protected in the sun for longer stretches of time. SPF protection is about the percentage of UV rays that are blocked from your skin, not how long they get blocked for. No matter which level of SPF you choose, it's wisest to reapply every two hours, or less if you have been swimming or sweating.

The good news is that sunscreens are pretty stable ingredients and can be easily mixed with other ingredients, like moisturizers and antioxidants. Woo hoo! Using an SPF lotion, cream, or gel to moisturize is a great way to use one product instead of two. And if you want to use a tinted sunscreen to give a sheer coverage to your skin, go for it. Not a thing wrong with multitasking like that.

JUST STOP depending on your makeup for your SPF protection. This is going to disappoint a lot of women out there, but it's literally impossible for makeup to contain creams, pigments, and enough sunscreen to give us the level of protection we really need. The amount of makeup you would have to wear to get the recommended level of sun protection is about ten times more than you would regularly wear. Think about that . . . ten times more makeup. That wouldn't look cute—not one little bit. SPF should always be applied separately, and any protection you get from your makeup is just a cherry on top.

Now, let's take the other fork in the skincare path and ease on down the road to hydration.

Hydrate, Hydrate, Hydrate—
Until You're Blue in the Face

Your face won't actually turn blue, but the punctuation mark on any skincare routine is applying moisturizer before you go to bed at night. Moisturizers are particularly effective at night when they soothe skin that's been irritated by all the many environmental factors we encounter each day. They can also soothe the skin when applied on top of the effective—but possibly irritating—treatment products we apply at night. Moisturized skin also looks plumper and smoother.

Is it absolutely necessary to use a separate moisturizer for eyes, face, neck, and body? Not necessarily, but I like to use one that's formulated specifically for the delicate area around the eyes. For everything else, one-stop shopping is Lazy Perfection approved.

> Okay. So just to recap. Your LAZY PERFECTION SIMPLE SKINCARE TRACK is:
> 1) Cleanse in p.m. for sure; in a.m. optionally
> 2) Treat with Retinols daily or as tolerated, AHAs three to four times per week, or a combination of both
> 3) Use SPF protection during the day
> 4) Moisturize at night

That doesn't seem so bad, right? Five minutes tops. Now if you're so inclined, you can step it up to the:

Lazy Perfection Sophisticated Skincare Track

This track includes all of the steps from the Simple Track, plus the introduction of a serum.

Serum Magic

"Serums" are quite possibly the most common vehicles for delivering specific skin-treating ingredients. They are lightweight and molecularly small, which enables them to literally stuff your skin with good ingredients that can get past the skin barrier into the deeper layers where they can be effective on a cellular level. I know it sounds like a science lesson, but all you need to remember is that serums should be applied immediately after washing or toning, and before any AHAs, Retinols, or other heavier skincare products that might block their access into the deeper realms. Serums go first because they need to have access to the deeper layers of the skin, sunscreen gets applied at the very end, just before makeup, since it's your last line of defense against UV damage.

This is the ideal point in your skincare routine to start looking at your complexion in an objective way and identify what it is you want to treat. Remember how exfoliation is Clueless Perfection because you don't really need to identify the specific issues you want to treat? Well, in selecting your serum, you need to give it just a little more thought.

Close your eyes and think of your Skincare Intention—you want to add a serum with one or all the following properties:

- Antioxidants—Antioxidants (the most common of which are vitamin A, C, and E, green tea, caffeine, resveratrol, and berries) protect our skin cells from something called *free radical damage*, aka destructive oxidization. Basically, free radical damage occurs as a consequence of exposure to the sun and pollution—essentially everything we live and breathe. Free radicals break down our skin's elastin and reduce our collagen production, leading to fine lines, wrinkles, and a dull tone. Free radicals suck.

- Peptides (aka amino acids)—Peptides are chains of amino acids that bind moisture and help to regenerate the skin by stimulating collagen growth. The jury is still out on exactly how effective they are, but they are purported to be helpful with softening the appearance of fine lines and wrinkles.

- Epidermal growth factors—EGFs are cells in our skin that basically act like tiny paramedics. When there's a trauma to the skin, like a burn, sun damage, fine lines, acne scars, EGFs speed the healing process by repairing and rejuvenating the tissue. They work especially well when you pair them with exfoliants, since removing dead skin cells leaves the EGFs easier access for deeper penetration.

- Arbutin, licorice root, kojic acid—These are also antioxidants, but they are generally used to prevent the formation of melanin by lightening and brightening dark spots and acne scars on the skin.

- Hyaluronic acid—Intensely hydrating and plumping, hyaluronic acid occurs naturally in the skin and binds up to one thousand times its own weight in water. Since our own production of it slows down over time, hyaluronic acid can give a big boost of hydration and add a plumping effect. Your moisturizer may have hyaluronic acid in it, and that's great, but in a serum formulation it'll have better access to the deeper layers of your skin where it can plump from underneath.

You can use serums with a single ingredient as a stand-alone treatment, or choose a multipurpose serum that addresses more than one skincare concern. Sometimes the ingredients will be listed right there on the label, and other times you have to look for key words like *hydrating, firming, plumping, smoothing, tightening, brightening, reparative,* or *rejuvenating* to help identify which one will meet your specific needs. The ones that say "Anti-Aging" are usually multipurpose and address a range of concerns.

Just remember—serums need to have direct access to the skin without anything heavy blocking their way.

Let me sum up your LAZY PERFECTION SOPHISTICATED SKINCARE TRACK:

1) Cleanse every night and in the morning if it helps
2) Apply serum a.m., p.m., or both, per the directions on the product
3) Use SPF protection during the day
4) Treat with Retinols, AHAs, or both
5) Moisturize at night

Lazy Perfection Sexy Skincare Track

Now we can start to think about putting on our GAME FACE in the LAZY PERFECTION SEXY SKINCARE TRACK. This is the bonus step for anyone who has the time, energy, or budget available to add in-office cosmetic or aesthetic services into their routine. These services might feel like they're a game, all luxury and pampering, but they can give you transformation-level results.

Some of those services might include:

- Traditional facials WITHOUT aggressive extractions, please—those can scar and inflame your skin! Gentle extractions are okay, as long as they don't make your eyes water in pain or leave you wounded!

- Aggressive exfoliation treatments like prescription-strength AHAs, dermaplaning, microdermabrasion or chemical peels to smooth and brighten the complexion and speed cell turnover

- Radiofrequency or ultrasonic treatment for skin tightening

- Collagen repair treatments like microneedling or intensive pulse light therapy (IPL)

- Resurfacing, scar removal, and sun damage treatments like lasers
- Neuromodulators, such as Botox to freeze muscles and smooth fine lines
- Fillers to smooth the appearance of deeper lines and wrinkles

At the end of the day, no matter whether you are getting in-office services or are treating your skin at home, consistency is key. In-office services will likely resolve specific issues faster than home products can, but what you do at home is every bit as important and will get you visible results over time.

Putting a Smile on Your Face

If I were the boss of your face and was in control of allocating your skincare dollars for Sexy Skincare Track in-office or spa services, here's the way I would prioritize them, from most important to least—and I know the results would put a smile on your face because this is the way I approach my own skincare.

- Monthly or seasonal prescription strength exfoliation facials or peels for faster cell turnover. This will keep your skin feeling smooth and looking bright and help your at-home skincare program work more efficiently and effectively. Plus, they are relatively fast services that require no downtime.

- Minimal Botox or fillers one to two times per year to smooth fine lines and improve the appearance of skin laxity. The more you do these treatments now, the less you need to do later because they give your skin a break from the natural aging process, allowing new lines to form more slowly. I don't advocate overdoing it—a little is enough and being totally frozen looks ridiculous—and my recommendation comes with a warning. Botox and fillers are a slippery slope—if you treat just one area, you are likely to notice the flaws in other areas much more acutely.

- Collagen repair treatments like microneedling to stimulate your own collagen and elastin production, giving you longer-term improvements in skin barrier function, tightness, and smoothing. Most dermatologists or spas recommend a series of these treatments, but the results after just one are pretty great.
- Radiofrequency/ultrasonic treatments if skin laxity on the jawline, neck, and eyes REALLY bothers you. Some of these treatments have only subtle results; some are quite painful; and most of them require a series of treatments to see longer-term benefits. Costs can be high, so you have to be prepared to make an investment and then maintain any results you see with regular follow-up services.
- Lasers—OF COURSE if you have acne or other scarring and have struggled with associated skin-self-esteem issues, you should move this up to the top of your priorities list. Restoring a smooth skin texture can actually be life-changing.
- Traditional facials—Surprised I put them as so low on this list? I have to confess that they are not my fave. 1) They are time-consuming compared to exfoliating facials and 2) you get much more tangible and longer-lasting results from an exfoliating facial. Sure, a traditional facial makes your skin look hydrated and soft, but as soon as you wash your face or work out, it pretty much goes back to the way it looked before. If you enjoy being pampered and find it relaxing, then by all means, enjoy.

Face of an Angel

In conclusion, if you want the face of an ageless, flawless, heavenly being, then you have to be good to your skin and create a consistent routine using the right types of products and treatments for your particular skin type. Your reward is likely to be more youthful-looking skin for an eternity, or at least a few decades!

CHAPTER FIVE

Game, Set, and Makeup Match

IT'S TIME TO PUT INTO PRACTICE ALL THE STEPS WE'VE TALKED about. So far you've:

- Cleaned out your old makeup
- Set your Beauty Intention
- Decided what you want your "look" to be
- Are armed with all the information you need to get out there and purchase what you need for your new Lazy Perfection Look
- Figured out your skincare routine

You're all warmed up, ladies, and it's time to take a swing at your new, updated, Lazy Perfection Look and Track. I know you can do it! Waiting to take the court . . . your complexion products . . . Primer, Foundation, Concealer, and Powder.

I've said it before and I'll say it again: if you don't have perfect skin, *you can fake it.* In fact, I'll take it one step further and say that if you need to you *should* fake it. Because guess what, folks? Pretty skin makes everything else look pretty, too. It's called "foundation" for a reason. The way your skin looks lays the groundwork for all your other makeup. It sets the tone for the rest of your face. It's the foundation on which everything else is built.

And since we don't want your foundation to settle or get cracked, and we do want it to look fresh, hydrated, and smooth, I am going to help you figure out the best products for you and how to apply them.

Quit Being Such a B-Word (and It's Not Ball Boy)

Blotches and Blemishes . . . they are some serious Bad Bs, if you know what I mean. And Undereye Bags, and Big Pores . . . they're Bs, too.

Thank goodness for the B-Slayers—Primer, Foundation, Concealer, and Powder. Superheroes, all. These are the products you need to get your skin looking even, smooth, youthful, and fresh. You don't have to use them all at the same time if you don't want to, but if you don't like what Mother Nature gave you . . . or has done to you over the years . . . just remember, it's totally possible to fake pretty skin.

First Serve—Primer

There's some controversy in the makeup artistry community about primer and whether it's really necessary. Purists say that they don't like to put anything between the skin and the makeup, but let me tell you the purposes primers serve, and then you can decide for yourself whether or not it is something you want to add to your routine.

- If you have a problem with your makeup fading over the course of the day, a basic primer creates a barrier that prevents absorption into the skin. This issue generally applies to women who have drier skin.

- If you find that your skin gets oily and your makeup starts to slide and get shiny, a mattifying primer creates a barrier that prevents the oils in your skin from surfacing and disturbing your makeup.

- If you have enlarged pores or small fine lines that your makeup settles into, a primer can fill the empty spaces to create an even, smooth surface onto which your makeup can evenly glide.

- If your skin tone is dull or lackluster, or you have lots of sun spots, primers that illuminate have subtle reflective properties that bounce the light away from your skin, making any flaws less visible.

- If you have redness or uneven coloration in your skin, color-correcting primers can balance out discoloration and create the illusion of even tone. A word of warning about color-correcting primers . . . only use them where you need them. If you apply them where you don't need them, you're going to end up looking, well, discolored.

Primers often contain silicone or dimethicone, both of which swell when they come in contact with oils, which is what keeps your makeup intact. You know the way you check the ingredients listed on your foods? You can do the same with your makeup. The "cones" will be listed right there for you to see. There are a couple of things to be aware of when it comes to the "cones" . . .

If your skin is dry, there's no oil to be absorbed, which can lead to the primer balling up and creating a lumpy mess when you put on your makeup. That's just annoying.

If your skin is sensitive or reactive, silicones and dimethicones can be irritating, so it's better to avoid them.

Tournament Ready

Now we're ready to talk about the makeup star all-star: foundation. Foundation evens out your skin tone, diffuses the appearance of flaws and makes everything look smooth and fresh, but when it comes right down to it, it can make or break your whole beauty look.

JUST STOP thinking that any old foundation will do as long as your color looks even. Texture and finish are every bit as important as color and have to work with your particular skin type.

In chapter 3, I outlined some basic vocabulary terms for you related to the CONSISTENCY, COVERAGE, and FINISH of your products, but here's an easy chart for you to help determine the type of foundation that will be best for you.

	MATTE/ VELVET	SATIN	ILLUMINATING	DEWY	TINTED MOISTURIZER	CREAM TO POWDER/ MINERAL POWDER
	Medium to Full Coverage	Light to Full Coverage	Sheer to Medium Coverage	Light to Medium Coverage	Sheer to Light Coverage	Medium to Full Coverage
Normal	x	x	x	x	x	x
Dry		x	x	x	x	
Combination	x	x			x	x
Oily	x					x
Fine Lines		x	x	x	x	
Discoloration	x	x	x			x

Match Point

The number one, most important factor when you're matching your foundation color is to make 100 percent for damn sure that your face, neck, and chest are all the same color. It's the only way you can truly win at the game of foundation. You must match.

We've all seen women who have a line around their cheek or jaw that's not at all the same color as their neck or chest. It's a distraction, no? And don't we judge the wearer when we see that? Just a little bit? It is, I remind you, human nature to judge, and while of course we know that mismatched or unblended foundation doesn't make the wearer a bad person, it certainly doesn't make her TPW. You can never even tell whether TPW is wearing foundation, which is the mark of an excellent foundation selection. Just another way in which she is admirable.

For the rest of us—even me, getting the ideal color match of foundation to your skin, can be really, really tricky. Sometimes it depends on the eye of the sales associate helping you, sometimes it depends on the lighting in the store, and in cases where you can't try it on before making your purchase because the packaging is sealed or you've selected it online, it depends on a certain amount of dumb luck. So here are a few ways you can mitigate the likelihood of losing the match:

When trying on foundation in a department or specialty store, draw a small line of makeup vertically along your jawline and down onto your neck. If it disappears into your skin, it is the right one for you. Simple. Lazy Perfection.

JUST STOP using your forehead to match your foundation. The objective is to make sure that your face, neck, and chest are in sync, so it's not going to be helpful to assess color based on the area of your face that's the farthest away from your neck and chest. The same goes for matching foundation on your inner wrist or hand—it's likely a much lighter color than your face.

If you're not able to try on the makeup because it's in a sealed package, you can get a fairly good idea about whether a color will work for you by facing a mirror and holding the bottle at arm's length, roughly around the height of your cheeks, and then squinting through one eye. I'm not kidding. Better to look ridiculous now than when you have mismatched coloring on your face and your neck! If the bottle sort of disappears in your line of vision, then you know you are in the right color ballpark.

If you are buying foundation (or any makeup) online, sight unseen, then you can look up swatches—stripes of product to show color, coverage, and finish—on the Internet. The best bloggers will have pictures of the swatches shot in natural light, indoor light, on their own face, in layers, and in a lineup with other foundations so you can see how they compare and contrast. *The Beauty Look Book, The RAEviewer, Beauty Professor,* and *Temptalia* are my go-tos.

Once you decide to try out a foundation, checking the color match in natural light will give the truest read. So get near a window or better yet, step outside. If that's not a possibility, then hold a handheld mirror above your head and look up into it. This will block out the fluorescent lights and give you a better idea of whether it matches. It will also help you determine whether the texture is suitable for your skin. Has it settled into your pores or fine lines? Grabbed on to any little dry patches? Changed color on your skin (called oxidizing)? No matter what type of foundation you use, it should not be visible to the untrained eye and should meld seamlessly with your skin. Like TPW's always does.

A word about oxidizing: When foundations change color on the skin, deepening either within minutes or hours to an orangey tone, it's because they are out of balance with the pH in your skin. Using a primer will help to prevent it from happening, but at the end of the day, what works on your friend may turn an odd shade of orange on you. And, unfortunately, there's no way to tell other than to try. Which is why I always suggest my Lazy Perfection Three-Day Rule.

Foundation needs three days to prove itself to you. Sometimes it takes that long to see how it wears in different environments/climates, different lighting, how it looks on camera, and, most importantly, whether it irritates your skin or causes breakouts. Most department and specialty stores will provide samples with enough to last you a few days. If you like it, you can either pop back to the store or order online since you'll already know exactly what you need.

Pep Rally

We need to talk about something I call the Cosmetic Continuum. All your makeup lives side by side and works together, with small variables having little impact on the overall effect of the look. But this is where we need to consider the seasonality of foundation. The bottom line is that there are some small adjustments that should be made to account for changes in our skin due to weather.

JUST STOP thinking that one foundation will work for you year-round. Purchase the same one in two different shades that you can mix, match, and layer as your skin color naturally adjusts and when seasons change.

To account for spring and summer, your foundation should be lighter in texture but slightly deeper in color. If you don't want to buy a whole new foundation for summer, then a simple way to make it wear better on your skin is to lighten up your moisturizer. For example, you can step down from a cream to a lotion, which is thinner and lighter, or from a lotion to a gel, which provides even less surface hydration. The goal is to ensure that your makeup doesn't slip and slide on warm skin or crack and crease on cold skin.

No Advantage

When it comes to actually applying your foundation, there really are no rules. This attitude is not going to make me popular with sales associates who want to sell you foundation brushes, but truthfully—and despite the fact that I have my own line of Lazy Perfection makeup brushes—the only things that matter when you apply your foundation are that it feels comfortable and is easy to do, and that it ends up well-blended, whether you use your fingers, a sponge or a brush.

Having said that, certain types of foundation do work better with certain tools, so here are some handy little tips to keep in mind when you're looking for an application advantage.

- LIQUIDY foundations, including serum formulas, the ones that you can shake and hear sloshing around in their container, are best applied with a sponge. They are such thin formulas that they streak easily, and having little bristle tracks or finger sweeps on your skin is the opposite of invisible makeup. Alternately, you can apply them with your fingers or a brush, and then lightly pat over them with a slightly damp sponge to smooth out any streaks left behind.

- CREAMY foundations, the ones that have a slightly thick, buttery texture are the most versatile as they apply well with fingers, a sponge, or a brush. However, if you choose to apply with a sponge, a damp sponge will give you the most natural-looking result as it adds hydration into your skin at the same time as it presses in the makeup.

- STICK foundations have a solid, dense texture that can be either swiped directly onto the skin and then blended with fingers or a sponge, or can be swept into with fingers or a brush that then goes onto the skin.

- POWDER OR MINERAL POWDER foundations get the best application results if you apply with a densely packed brush. They need heat and friction in order to meld into the skin, and a light, fluffy brush simply doesn't have the power to do it.

- CREAM-TO-POWDER foundation is designed for oily or combination skin, so that it glides onto the skin but then dries to a powdery, long-wear finish. A dense, flat brush or sponge are the most effective tools for this type of foundation.

Fault!

Fully realizing that a tennis analogy is not what one would ordinarily find in a book about beauty, it just fits so well here, I have to go with it. It gives a little sporty flavor to balance out all the pretty, pretty makeup talk, don't you think?

Okay. So. You know that when a tennis serve lands in the wrong box, it's called a fault and play can't continue, right? Concealer is a surefire way to make sure you never serve a fault. You are serving up a can of concealer whoop-ass, and it's your flaws that get defeated.

If I were playing tennis in the glaring midday sun, all eyes on me, the first thing I would do, right after applying my SPF and donning a hat to prevent sun damage (obvi), would be to cover up my undereye circles. Seriously, those circles should never see the light of day. For many of us, they are our most troublesome fault.

Concealer can be used for a whole lot more than just covering up undereye circles though. You can use it to fill in enlarged pores; even out redness; cover up broken capillaries, veins, or dark spots; lift your mouth and eyes; sculpt the shape of your brows and lips; and correct small makeup mishaps.

Accurate Aim

In my experience, trying to find the right concealer is a bit like being run ragged by an opponent who has more accurate aim than you. There are SO many options, both in type and color; it can be exhausting trying to determine the right shade. I can't even count how many lines carry products with the word *beige* in it . . . and every single one of those beiges is different— Gah! No joke—if someone can tell me the difference between sand beige, medium beige, and warm beige, I will give you the keys to my car.

I'm going to make things really simple when it comes to selecting your color. You've swatched and chosen your foundation, now, there's just one simple step left between you and Lazy Perfection Concealing. Go ahead and reswatch your foundation color—or hold it at arm's length in front of the mirror with your sexy squint going on—and then swatch or hold the concealer next to it.

- For undereyes—your concealer should be a little lighter than your foundation.

- For blemishes or discoloration on the skin—your concealer should be the identical color as your foundation, or a teensy bit darker.

And that's really and truly all there is to it. Sounds almost too easy, right? I'm going to make it even easier.

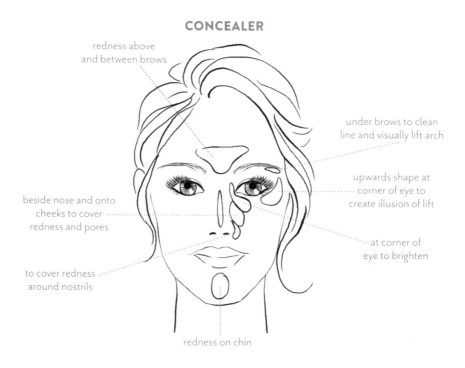

CONCEALER

redness above and between brows

under brows to clean line and visually lift arch

upwards shape at corner of eye to create illusion of lift

beside nose and onto cheeks to cover redness and pores

at corner of eye to brighten

to cover redness around nostrils

redness on chin

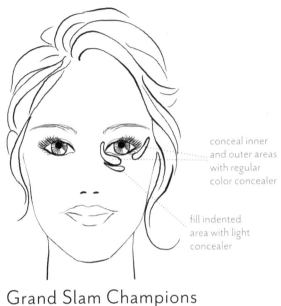

conceal inner
and outer areas
with regular
color concealer

fill indented
area with light
concealer

Grand Slam Champions

Makeup lines that have ten, twelve, or more color options still only have three to four best-sellers because they're the ones that are the most versatile across a range of skin tones. You can always ask a sales associate—in person or by phone—to share their best-selling colors, and once you make your purchase, you'll be able to see right away how it matches up with your foundation. I'll bet dollars to doughnuts that one of those best-sellers will work for you. That's why they're champions.

But . . . now there's this whole new world of color correcting that's become a mainstream phenom. I have to tell you, using pink, lavender, orange, red, and green is advanced artistry stuff and not really Lazy Perfection approved.

However (could you tell that was coming?), there is a Lazy Perfection color-correcting methodology for more common issues like pimples or deep, dark circles. There are only two things to keep in mind:

• If you have redness or blemishes on your skin, a yellow-based color will offset it. Think of yellow-based colors like banana slices for very fair skin, pita chips or hummus for light to medium skin, or peanut butter or cappuccino for medium to darker tones.

• If you have purplish discoloration like very dark undereye circles, scars or bruises, a peach-based color will neutralize the purple/blue/gray tones. Think peach sorbet for fair skin, cantaloupe or glazed doughnuts for light to medium skin, and pretzels or sweet potato chips for medium to darker tones.

Different formulas are going to be better for different purposes, so here's a handy dandy little chart for you to figure out what might work for you. You will undoubtedly realize I am hungry as I write this.

SKIN TONE	YELIOW UNDERTONES FOR COVERING REDNESS	PEACH TONE FOR COVERING PURPLE/GRAY/BLUE
FAIR	Banana Slices	Peach Sorbet
LIGHT	Pita Chips	Glazed Doughnut
LIGHT/MEDIUM	Hummus	Cantalope
MEDIUM	Coffee Ice Cream	Pretzels
MEDIUM/DARK	Peanut Butter	Roasted Almonds
DARK	Mocha Frappucino	Sweet Potato Chips

Here's a helpful tip about skintone . . . if you're wondering whether you're cool or warm, just remember that warm colors show up in a fire and cool colors show up in water and ice. You can always do the jewelry test to figure it out—If you look great in silver, you're cool; if gold flatters you more, you're warm. If you wear both colors well, congratulations, you're neutral.

Your Equipment

There are several ways to apply concealer—with a brush, a sponge, your fingers, or directly from the container. And once again, there is no right or wrong way—it all depends on you, your comfort level, and getting a well-blended result.

- Brushes have the advantage of being able to smooth or buff a smaller amount of product over a larger area, which means longer wear time and less likelihood of creasing or creeping. This is my personal preference. Use a tiny, pinpoint brush to cover small pimples and blemishes; a long, flat brush to smooth over pores and textural variances; and a soft domed-shaped brush to lightly buff over areas of discoloration.

JUST STOP applying dispenser-tip concealers directly onto your face. Whether they have a brush or a sponge built right in, it's difficult to control the amount of product that you click or twist up, which can result in over-, or underapplying. Plus, those brushes tend to be too skinny to get a smooth, even blend. You'll get much more control over how much concealer you apply and a prettier application if you either dab it onto your face and then blend with a brush, fingers, or a sponge, or dab it onto the back of your hand before applying it to your face with a brush, sponge, or finger.

- Fingers use body heat and friction to meld the concealer into the skin, giving a seamless look. Caveat—it's easy to tug or pull on the skin when using your fingers to apply, so a soft tapping motion with your ring finger is the gentlest approach to avoid overstretching the delicate skin around the eyes.

JUST STOP dragging the skin down when you apply undereye concealer. Not only are you messing with the delicate elastins in this thin skin area, but you are also increasing the likelihood of creasing. The second you stop stretching your skin, it bounces back to where it naturally rests, taking your concealer with it where it will settle into fine lines.

- As with fingers, sponges are effective for tapping concealer into the skin and are particularly helpful when covering a blemish as it can soften the edges of the applied area to make it fade more seamlessly into the rest of your skin.
- When applying directly from the container onto the skin, blending is still required to make it meld with the skin, and you can choose any of the above tools, based on your personal preference.

Here's a nifty little trick: if you apply your undereye concealer in a deep V-shape under your eyes, it doubles as a highlighter, brightening your cheeks and your whole complexion.

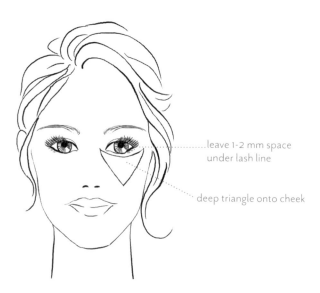

leave 1-2 mm space under lash line

deep triangle onto cheek

I have to admit that I am not a big fan of powder. If you are prone to shine, get oily, need to set blemish concealer in place, or have an event where long-wear is especially important, then it can be very useful and effective, but my Lazy Perfection Powder approach is to apply ONLY where needed.

I don't advocate powdering all over the face and dulling your natural sheen as a necessary last step in the process. That little bit of glow is what keeps us looking fresh and young, and besides, if you've applied primer, it should be helpful in many of the same ways powder is, preventing oils from surfacing or makeup from fading.

If you have skin that errs on the dry side, then powder is definitely not your friend. It'll just accentuate fine lines and dry patches. The Lazy Perfection objective is to look natural and fresh, and powder often doesn't play by the Lazy Perfection rules.

JUST STOP thinking that powder products are the best option for warm weather. It may seem that they would be, since powders absorb shine, but when we produce more oil than usual and add powder on top, all we've actually done is taken the first steps on the road to a "cakey" face by combining oil and flour.

There are two basic types of powder—pressed and loose. Pressed is far more convenient for travel as you are unlikely to have it leave your makeup bag covered with a layer of fine dust, but loose powder lasts longer because you need less of it, and it blends more smoothly and evenly on the skin because it's more finely milled (meaning that it's been ground into smaller particles).

And there are two schools of thought on powder color. You can use a translucent powder (aka "colorless" or "invisible," but looks white to the naked eye) or one that matches your foundation/skin. Honestly, I could go either way here, but am issuing a Lazy Perfection Warning to anyone with skin that's medium to dark. What's invisible on fair, light, or medium skin will not be invisible on you and can make you look like you just finished cleaning out a fireplace, with your face. Looking ashy isn't cute.

Regardless of the color you choose, the key to successful powder application is just one thing—your brush. In order to get a soft, natural, non cakey application of powder, your brush needs to be soft, fluffy, and flexible. When a brush is dense and rough, it picks up too much product from the pan, and makes it more challenging—and time-consuming—to blend. A soft brush collects less product and subtly whispers it onto your face.

> JUST STOP thinking that any old powder brush will do. Brushes for mineral powder or powder foundation need to be more dense and firm than brushes for loose or pressed powder so that they can build up the friction and heat needed to meld the makeup into the skin.

I am going on record as saying that I do not, in any way, advocate the use of the powder puffs or sponges that come with compact powders. There really should be a written contract for you to sign, swearing that you will throw it away once it becomes so filthy that the original surface of it is no longer visible. How many have I confiscated from my clients and thrown away? More than I can count. All they do is pack makeup onto your skin and carry the leftover creams and oils from your face back into the pan, which then build up on the makeup and eventually make it work less effectively. And don't even get me started on the hygiene issues here. Blech.

The Ball's in Your Court

Remember, you can mix and match the SIMPLE, SOPHISTICATED, and SEXY Lazy Perfection techniques to find the one that's best for you. Lazy Perfection is not about HAVE TOs or SHOULDs. It's about finding a look that works HOLISTICALLY for your skin type, your technical application skills, your personal style, and your lifestyle.

Simple

Perfect for: When you're running late; a day at work where you won't see clients or customers; weekend brunch; coffee with a friend; exhausted moms; women who don't like a lot of makeup; lazy days

PRIMER—Totally optional

FOUNDATION—Sheer- to light- coverage tinted sunscreen or tinted moisturizer, applied with fingers and blotted with sponge, if necessary, to remove excess on the surface and set the rest in place

CONCEALER—Under inner and outer corners of eyes and lightly blended onto any areas of discoloration or enlarged pores on the nose and sides of nose/inner cheeks, between the eyebrows, on the chin, and possibly on the eyelids

JUST STOP Concealer should never be applied all the way up to the lower lash line and be in contact with the roots of your lashes, as it wipes out the natural shading and makes the eyes look smaller. Always leave a couple of millimeters unconcealed.

POWDER—Totally optional

Sophisticated

Perfect for: When you need a little extra wear time; meetings or presentations at work; a casual date or event; meetings at your child's school; casual lunch with a colleague or friend; career women; moms who have a few minutes to spend on makeup; women who only like a little makeup but want to look put together

> **PRIMER**—Spread a thin layer with fingers
>
> **FOUNDATION**—Light to medium coverage as daylight and fluorescent office/school lighting can make heavier coverage appear obvious, applied with tool of choice
>
> **CONCEALER**—Dot undereyes in inner and outer corners only, then blend together; using long/flat brush, sweep into arch of brow to sculpt and define the shape (makes the eyes look more open); use blending or pinpoint brush to spot-cover blemishes on the skin and any areas of redness or discoloration
>
> **POWDER**—Optional—lightly dusted over areas that tend to get oily/shiny and to set any blemish concealer in place

Sexy

Perfect for: Date night; dinner with friends; a special event; an important presentation at work; when long-wear is required; when your photograph is being taken; women who like a little more coverage; women who want to step up their makeup look

PRIMER—Illuminating primer is great for evening so you can to attract any available light in a darkly lit room to your face. Spread a thin layer with fingers

FOUNDATION—Medium to full coverage, applied with tool of choice and blotted with damp sponge to set into place

CONCEALER—Apply undereyes in deep V shape from inner to outer corner to brighten and bring highlight to cheek area, additional spot coverage as needed, under arch of brows, drawn up diagonally with long, flat brush at corners of eyes and corners of lips to give appearance of lift (make sure to pat/blend away edges), at edge of the bottom lip to define and sharpen

POWDER—Lightly dust on top of any area where concealer was applied. I rarely powder under my eyes. But if you want to ensure that your concealer doesn't crease, save the undereye area for last when there is almost no powder left on the brush. Too much powder under the eyes looks dry and aging.

Congratulations, you Lazy Perfection player! You're getting the swing of things now!

CHAPTER SIX

Eyes on the Prize

TPW IS BEWILDERING, NO? SHE'S THE KIND OF WOMAN WHO MAKES it all seem . . . just easy. Everything about her is put together and lovely, but if you look carefully, her beauty emanates mostly from her eyes. Not only are they kind and interested, they are framed by thick dark lashes that look fluffy, soft, and überfeminine.

Windows to the Soul

When you ask someone the first feature they notice on someone's face, it's almost always the eyes. You can gauge so much about a person based on her eyes—they hold so much expression. But the eyes are also the first feature to show signs of age because the thin, delicate skin around them can betray an otherwise youthful, fresh complexion.

I've worked with thousands of women, talking to them about their makeup struggles. And if you ask any of them the hardest part of her makeup routine—the part they feel the least confident about—nine times out of ten, the answer will be the eyes. I mean, it makes perfect sense—they've got very little surface area but have an enormous impact.

That's stressful. Now, that's not to say that the eyes always have to be the "Star of the Show"—but even if they are simply a supporting cast member, they can ruin an otherwise delightful production number by distracting our attention with clumpy lashes, creased shadow, or eyeliner that's tried to break away and get to center stage . . . or at least the center of the face. The eyes always seem to pull focus, for better or for worse.

Easy on the Eyes

So many women seem to have this notion that in order for them to look "done" they need to follow some prescribed path that's been in place since the dawn of time . . . or at least since the dawn of eye shadow. But I'm sure you can guess my take on it. I say, it's okay to be lazy about your eye makeup because you can still easily get a gorgeous look.

There are four key areas to figuring out how to make the most of your eyes:

• Understanding your shape and making it work for you

• Finding the most flattering colors and textures

• Being honest with yourself about your technical skill set and what level of detail you can realistically achieve

• Using the tools that will simplify and streamline your application process

JUST STOP thinking that you need to use every shadow in the palette, or any at all. Simple eye makeup can be every bit as dramatic and impactful as a four-step eye shadow application, and skipping eye shadow altogether in favor of liner and mascara is always a fine option.

Eye of the Beholder

So, the first thing you want to consider is the shape of your eyes, because the fact of the matter is that your particular eye shape is not going to be right for every style of application. It isn't all universally doable, or universally flattering. But, if you can learn the techniques and make choices that flatter your eyes, then your time will be well spent.

Take a look at this chart and see if you can spot yourself.

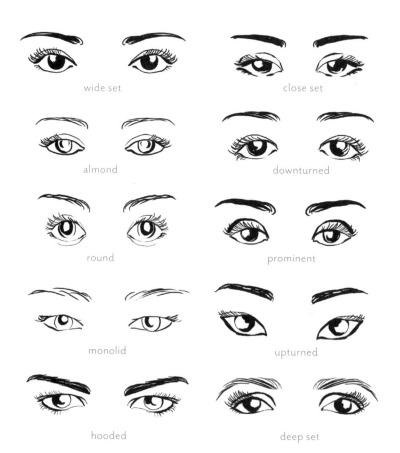

wide set   close set

almond   downturned

round   prominent

monolid   upturned

hooded   deep set

Still not sure? Allow me to break this down into three simple points.

1) There are two basic eye shapes:

- **Round**—Look straight ahead. If you can see the very edge of the rim of your iris, you have round eyes.

- **Almond**—Look straight ahead. If the rims of your iris aren't visible, then they are almond-shaped. Also, if they look like they're the same shape as an almond, obviously.

2) There are several different placements of eyes on the face:

- **Wide Set**—If there is enough space between your eyes to add a whole other eye, then you are wide set.

- **Close Set**—The exact opposite of wide-set eyes, close-set eyes have less than an eye's width between them.

- **Deep Set**—Deep-set eyes have the appearance of a prominent brow bone and a recessed lid. If you can rest your index finger vertically on your brow bone and then flatten it on your cheek without coming in contact with the lid, your eyes are deep set.

- **Upturned**—Hold an eyeliner pencil horizontally across the center of your eye. If the outer corners slant up, your eyes are upturned.

- **Downturned**—Hold an eyeliner pencil horizontally across the center of your eye. If the corners point down, you guessed it—you have downturned eyes.

3) And finally, there are several different lid structures.

- **Monolid**—If you have no crease at all, your shape is monolid.

- **Hooded**—If little to none of your lid is visible when your eyes are open, you are hooded. Some people are born hooded; others become hooded over time.

- **Prominent**—Looks just like it sounds—your lid pops forward a little. This feature is most commonly found with round eyes.

Some women are straight-up almond or round while others have mixins like round and protruding, almond and hooded, round and close set, almond and wide set, and downturned, etc. Almond is far and away the most common shape, whether downturned, upturned, or hooded.

So what does this all mean for you? Well, there are certain ways to place your eye shadow and eyeliner that can either enhance or take away from your eyes.

Bull's-Eye

Knowing where to aim your makeup so that you can get it in just the right place every time is crucial to the success of a Lazy Perfection eye makeup application.

For the purpose of mapping out your eye makeup application, think of the eyes as being broken into thirds:

- The inner white of the eye
- The iris
- The outer white of the eye

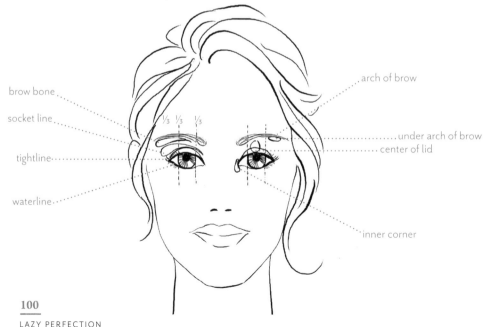

And here are the key anatomical features you need to know:

- **Tightline**—This is the underside of your upper lash line, where the roots of your lashes meet the fleshy, pale skin underneath them.
- **Lid**—This is the largest area of your lid, the one that opens and closes.
- **Crease**—Where the skin on your lid folds, but this is not where you should be aiming placement of any of your shadows. The skin can move around under your brush, so it's better to aim for firmer ground (aka the socket line).
- **Socket line**—The true crease. This is the bony area that tracks along your eye socket, above your lid.
- **Brow bone**—This is the top, flat part of the eye socket, underneath your eyebrow.
- **Arch of the brow**—This is the flat bony area directly underneath the highest point of your eyebrows, on the outer one-third.
- **Waterline**—This is the pale fleshy area above your lower lash line. Where you probably applied too much black eyeliner when you were in high school.
- **Inner corner**—This is the small C-shaped area that hugs your tear duct.
- **Center of the lid**—When eyes are open and look straight ahead, the center of the lid is immediately above and in line with your iris, but below your socket line.

Bull's-eye. Now you know your target. But before we start with any makeup, we also need to understand our shadow, liner, and mascara options.

A Feast for the Eyes

There are thousands and thousands . . . and thousands . . . of different eye shadow, eyeliner, and mascara options out there. It's totally overwhelming. Choosing the right one can seem like a challenge greater than climbing Mount Everest backward and blindfolded.

But once you start to understand how it all breaks down, you'll be able to choose products that will work for you and not some idealized version of what you think you should be able to achieve.

So with eye shadows, there are four basic finishes, all of which can be found in powder or cream formulations:

- **Matte**—No shimmer at all. Great for very crepey lids, but can look chalky or flat.
- **Satin**—A hint of shimmer. Flattering on everyone due to its subtle brightening effect.
- **Shimmer**—Sparkly particles that are visible in the pan. Not super flattering on skin that is crepey as it can accentuate fine lines, or can "drop" onto the cheeks and settle in those fine lines.
- **Metallic**—Sparkle that has been so finely ground, it has a smooth, mirrored effect. Flattering on everyone when used strategically and/or in small doses.

And there are six basic eyeliners—

- **Pencil (waxy)**—Standard eye pencil texture. May or may not be water resistant or waterproof. May tug on the lash line during application, so not ideally suited for anyone with crepey skin or shaky hands.
- **Pencil (gel)**—A smooth, gliding texture. Generally water resistant. Relatively easy for anyone to apply and also works well for tightlining and for the waterline.

- Pencil (kohl)—A soft, powdery texture that smudges easily. Not truly waterproof, but water will roll over it without streaking. Great for a soft, smoky look.
- Powder—Wet or dry eye shadow applied along the lash line with a brush. Looks very natural and works on most women, although some women will smudge or fade more easily than others.
- Gel—Potted gel liner is generally waterproof and long-wearing. Works well for tightlining but requires some technical control and a suitable brush.
- Liquid—Comes in a pen with a sponge or brush tip that gives a precise application. It's best used either to thicken the appearance of the lash line or to create dramatic cat eye or graphic eye looks.

JUST STOP beating yourself up over not being able to apply liquid liner. It is the most technically challenging liner to apply as the thin consistency, thin tip, and wet finish require a steady hand and precise placement. For these reasons, liquid eyeliner is not Lazy Perfection approved.

And finally, when it comes to mascara, there are hundreds of thousands of different choices, but the bottom line, is that *there's no perfect mascara*. As long as it doesn't clump, smudge, or flake on you, then it's perfectly fine. Mascara is very individual. It's so much about your own body chemistry, there's no way to predict what sort of results you will get based on someone else's experience or recommendation. Which is why I wholeheartedly approve of drugstore mascara. Take the thirty-five dollars you were going to spend on one designer mascara and get yourself three or four drugstore ones instead. The chances are high that you'll land on one that works every bit as well.

Here are the basic types of mascara:

- **Lengthening**—This type of mascara places the product on each individual lash and combs it through from root to tip. You'll get defined, long lashes but not necessarily much thickness.
- **Volumizing**—This type of mascara is all about thickening up the lashes and making them look lush and dense. Volumizing applicators will be densely packed with bristles so that they can grab even your smallest lash hair and coat all the way around it.

- **Curling**—Not Lazy Perfection approved. I have yet to find a curling mascara that actually curls. If you want to lift the look of your lashes, work your volumizing mascara into the roots of your lashes and then lift them a bit and hold for a few seconds to set into place. Volumizing mascaras tend to be waxier than lengthening mascaras, which is why they work better for this lifting technique.
- **Tube**—Tube mascara is great for anyone with particularly wispy, short lashes. It grips on to the tip of the lash and basically shrink-wraps

around it, adding extended length to each individual follicle (but not a lot of volume). When you wash your face at the end of the day, you will see the little tips in your sink.

- Fiber—Fiber mascaras have small, powdery particles in them that coat the lashes in order to make them look thicker and fuller. They are either sold in a white base form, on top of which you apply your regular mascara, or with a pigment already mixed in. They aren't Lazy Perfection approved because they tend to cause a lot of clumping, which in turn takes a lot of time to correct. Plus, the little fibers can get into your eyes, and that's not comfortable.

JUST STOP listening to that old beauty myth about dusting powder on your lashes before applying mascara in order to thicken them. Powder is made to absorb oil, so while your lashes may look great at first, it will eventually suck away the moisture from your mascara, too, leaving you with a flaky mess.

Here are descriptions of the most common applicator shapes and what they can do for you.

Lengthening mascara wands have bristles that are placed far apart and can be as small as a nub. These are designed to move in a long, gliding motion so that the lashes get separated and then extended from root to tip. Lengthening mascara applicators are generally long and thin.

Volumizing mascara wands have lots of bristles, often in varying lengths, that are designed to grip firmly at the root of the lashes, grabbing even the smallest hairs, and giving them a 360-degree coverage. To apply volumizing mascara, gently press the applicator into the roots of the lashes and wiggle slightly from side to side before pulling through to the ends.

There are plenty of very gimmicky mascara wand shapes out there, promising all sorts of astonishing results, but at the end of the day, as long as you can recognize these basic shapes and know the result they will give, you'll be able to choose the one that's best for you.

A Sight for Sore Eyes

There are a couple of mascara warnings I feel I need to issue . . . First, waterproof formulas can be dry and brittle on the lashes and can actually cause some long-term damage. If you know you'll need extra wear time or tear-proof protection, try applying a regular mascara and then adding a coat of waterproof on top to seal it in.

If your eyes are sensitive and prone to irritation, look for mascaras that are both fragrance-free and hypoallergenic. It's often the fragrance in mascara that can cause redness and watering, or ingredients such as parabens and aluminum powder. You'll be able to find a list of ingredients on the mascara packaging.

And finally, make sure that your mascara comes off easily at the end of the day, with your regular face wash or an eye makeup remover. If you are losing multiple lashes when you take it off, it could be the sign of an allergy. And of course, having to vigorously rub at your eyes to get your mascara off is certainly not ideal.

More Than Meets the Eye

I don't dislike false eyelashes or eyelash extensions—I think they can look gorgeous, in fact. But they are not Lazy Perfection approved. Applying false lashes (individuals, flares, or strips) with glue is fussy and technical, and when done incorrectly, may not only look obvious and distort the shape of the eyes, but may also lead to irritation or even lash loss. If you're having your makeup done, go for it. Nothing says glamour more than a few falsies. But doing them at home daily is not at all lazy.

Semipermanent eyelash extensions are theoretically Lazy Perfection because once they are on you can skip mascara for weeks and wake up with long, dark lashes, However, they are high maintenance in their care and upkeep, and limiting in terms of other products you can or cannot use with them (like eyeliner or mascara), and they are expensive. Plus, as they fall out, you're left with little gaps in your lash line. Like hair extensions or false nails, they must be applied by a highly skilled and well-trained technician; otherwise, you may end up with permanent follicle damage, irritation, or, worst-case, a scratched cornea. Lots of women love them, but I don't believe that they are the quick, easy fix that so many believe them to be.

An easy interim step is a lash tint. They're especially great if your lashes are very pale, or if you are someone who has an aversion to mascara, but you should be sure that you are working with an experienced practitioner who will only use a natural, vegetable-based dye. You do not want chemical ingredients that close to your eyes.

Eyes Wide Open

I'm not going to advocate that you use lots of different shadows on your lids, because that would be antithetical to "Lazy Perfection," but there are some key placements and tricks you should know to make the most of your particular eye shape. For some of you, I will suggest focusing more on shadow application, for others a focus on liner and mascara. My goal in this chapter is to show you how to take simple but significant steps that will open wide the windows to your souls. And remember, you may fall into more than one of these categories, so you can consult the chart earlier in this chapter to gain even more clarity.

In the Eyes of the Gods

Thou shalt follow my Ten Lazy Perfection Eye Makeup Commandments.

1) Your lids always need to be primed, meaning a base layer on top of which all your other shadow should be applied. If you experience creasing, a primer will work the same way as a foundation primer, creating a barrier between your lid and your makeup and helping to lock your shadow, liner, and even mascara into place. Eyelashes produce sebums the same way our scalps do, but using primer will help control the slip and slide. If your lids are red, gray, or discolored, a tinted primer will neutralize the uneven pigmentation. Priming can be as simple as dusting a little bit of powder on to absorb oils and help the rest of your shadow glide and blend more easily.

2) Always tap excess shadow off your makeup brush before touching it to your eye. This not only prevents loose particles from dropping down onto the cheeks, it also keeps the layers of product sheer and natural. It is always easier to apply more and build your coverage gradually than it is to wipe makeup away.

3) Always blend shadows after you apply them for a soft and diffused effect. Unblended shadows look like makeup—but blended makeup looks simply like an enhancement of your natural lid.

4) Liners do not have to be applied in one smooth stroke. The easiest liner approach is to make short, flicky strokes back and forth along the lash line. If you can feel your lashes moving, you are in the right place. If your mascara doesn't hit right at the roots, it will make your lashes look disconnected from the rest of your lid, like they are floating.

5) When in doubt, smudge. It's far and away the most forgiving, softest, and subtlest look for liner. Don't like the way your liner went on? Soften it with a smudge brush. Apply your liner unevenly? Use a smudge brush to even it out. Feel like your liner looks harsh? Yep. You guessed it. Smudge. Feel free to even skip the liner pencil and just smudge on some eye shadow as liner. It's so easy to do and looks very feminine and soft. Smudging is the cornerstone of Lazy Perfection eye makeup.

6) If the skin on your lid is crepey, you are better off patting your shadow into place than sweeping back and forth as it can lead to creasing and settling. Select gel liner pencils instead of waxy ones—they glide across the skin without any tugging.

7) Whether your lid is crepey or not, when applying shadows into the socket line or outer corner, the skin underneath your brush should not move. Shadow will look softer and more natural if it is floated onto the skin rather than spread.

8) A small amount of taupe eye shadow or taupe eye pencil applied underneath the lower lash line will create the illusion of height to the eye. Translation—it makes your lower lash line look lower, so your lid looks taller. I know it's scary for a lot of women to use liner on their lower lash line, but I promise you, this is a subtle effect—and it really works.

9) Everyone looks good with a tightline. Use a waterproof pencil or a gel liner with a brush to work a dark liner (black, brown, gray, or navy) underneath the roots of the upper lashes. This makes the lashes look thicker and darker, defines the shape of your eye, and makes the

whites of the eyes look whiter. This can be done alone or in addition to other eyeliner.

10) If you wear liner in your waterline, it should ALWAYS ALWAYS ALWAYS be paired with some sort of soft, smudged liner under the lower lash line, even if it's simply a taupe color. Without that additional soft line underneath, the eyes will look closed up and small.

JUST STOP accepting accidentally smudged liner as your lot in life. If you suffer from runaway liner, then make sure to apply your primer all the way to the roots of your lashes to create an oil-resistant barrier. You can also try waterproof formulas or layering a powder liner on top of your pencil to give it more grip and staying power.

JUST STOP thinking that black liner is going to be the most flattering. On light eyes and fair skin, it can look harsh, and as we age, that hard line can call attention to our softening skin. Opt instead for brown, navy, grey or plum.

Catching Your Eye

Let's take a look at all the different eye shapes so that you can identify yours and learn how to work with it.

Almond

The most common and versatile of all eye shapes, almond eyes that are not upturned, downturned, monolid, or hooded can be made to look round or long, as you prefer.

To create a rounder shape:

• Apply a base color on the lid, then softly apply a slightly darker shadow in the socket line in a rainbow shape, taking care to connect the shadow to the upper/outer lash line.

- Apply mascara across the upper and lower lash lines, concentrating in the center of both the top and bottom lashes.
- Apply liner all the way across the upper lash line but only on the outer one-third of the lower lash line, blending well so the end of the line fades instead of coming to a blunt stop.

To accentuate the long, almond shape:

- Apply shadow on the entire lid and then apply a deeper shade onto the outer one-third of the lid and socket line, extending slightly past the last outer lash.
- Liner should be applied all the way across the upper lash line, extending slightly past the last lash on the upper, outer corner. Liner can be applied almost all the way across the lower lash line, ending just shy of the inner corner. Smudge to soften.
- For added detail, create a > shape of slightly darker shadow at the outer corner of the eye and then blend with your other shadows.

Round

It's difficult to make round eyes look anything other than round, but you can create the illusion of a little lift at the outer corner.

- Apply shadow on the lid, taking care to avoid anything too shimmery or reflective as this can give the appearance of protrusion. Add contour by applying a slightly deeper shade in the socket line with a rainbow motion.
- With a deeper color, create a small > just above the last few outer corner lashes, from the base of the lashes into the socket line, taking care to blend carefully so the color melds into the others.

- Liner should be applied on the upper lash line from almost all the way at the inner corner (but not all the way), giving it a slight lift at the outer corner, just above the very outer lash. It's easiest to see where to make the lift if you keep your eyes open a bit when placing it.
- Mascara should be applied to the whole upper lash line but pay special attention to the outer one-third of the lashes, lifting them up and out.
- Lower lash mascara should be concentrated only on the outer one-third of the lash line.

Wide Set

- The key to makeup for wide-set eyes is to make sure that they don't look as though they are being pulled farther apart.
- Liner should be placed all the way into the inner corner on the top lash line and thickened over the center one-third of the lid, if possible but not extended past the outer corner of the eye.
- Place a shadow on the lid and a slightly deeper shade into the center part of the socket line, diffusing lightly over the outer socket line with the very lightest touch. There should be no shadows applied directly on the outer corners of the eyes other than what gets blended there.
- Liner should be aimed all the way into the inner corner, like a line pointing the way in.
- Mascara should be focused on the center of the lashes to create the illusion of height instead of length.

Close Set

A total opposite to wide-set eyes, all the darkness on this eye shape should be focused on the outer one-third to create the impression that they are being pulled further apart.

- Apply a base lid color then a deeper a socket line color drawn out long over the socket and turning the corner at the outer edge in a > shape to join with the lash line.
- Using a darker color, create a > at the outer corner of the eye and blend out to diffuse and elongate.
- Use a light highlighting color at the inner corner of the eye and under the arch of the brow to attract light and create the illusion of space.
- Eyeliner should be drawn from the center one-third of the eye across the outer one-third of the eye, extending slightly past the last lashes. This line should be smudged, diffused, and slightly lifted/elongated.

Deep-Set

Deep-set eyes look even deeper set when paired with dark or dull shadows. Look for reflective finishes that draw the light to them and make them look brighter.
- Use the same application technique as round eyes, taking care not to overdo dark liner as this will make the eyes look even deeper set.

Upturned

Upturned eyes are rare and terribly exotic. To enhance their look:
- Apply a light-medium shadow all over the lid.
- Apply a medium to dark color on the outer one-half of the base lid, blending carefully.
- Apply liner to the outer one-half of the upper lash line and the outer one-third of the lower lash line.
- Apply mascara all across the upper lash line with a focus on the outer one-third of the upper and lower lashes.

Monolid

- Apply a sheer, satin color all over the lid.
- If desired, with eyes open and chin tilted up to stretch the lid, apply a medium-toned shadow into the socket line and just beneath it.
- Apply a thick swath of a deep shadow across the lid, just above the lash line, instead of eyeliner, starting in the center one-third of the eye and extending just past the outer one-third.
- Apply plenty of mascara.

Downturned

The main thing to keep in mind with downturned eyes is the location of the last few lashes on your upper lash line. These will be your "color-by-number" guides to creating the appearance of lift.

- Apply a sheer, satiny shadow all over your lid and under the arch of the brow.
- With the eyes open, apply a medium to deep shade of eye shadow on the outer one-third of the lid, aiming to stay within the line of the last lashes on the upper/outer lash line. Extending past those lashes will pull the appearance of the corners down farther. This shadow should be aimed up toward the temples, in line with the outer tail of your eyebrow.
- Eyeliner applied on the upper lash line and lower lash line should not connect at the corner. Leave a small gap between them so that the eyes look more open and upturned.
- If you are not able to get the lift in your shadow or liner application, take a damp Q-tip, hold it inside the very outer corner of your eye—where your upper and lower lashes meet—and lightly sweep upward to pull your makeup up and into place.
- Apply mascara across the entire lash line and in the center of the lower lash line.

Hooded

This is going to be an opinion in contrast to the one you hooded girls have probably heard for years, but I don't see the point in struggling to apply detailed eye shadow on hooded eyes when the lid and crease are hardly even visible. Instead, I believe that the Lazy Perfection emphasis on hooded eyes should be on the lash line and lashes.

- Apply a light, satin finish color to the base lid, particularly on the inner corner of the eye since it's the most visible part.
- If you want to apply a deeper color shadow in the socket line, do it while your eyes are open and your chin is lifted slightly. This will stretch your lid so that your socket line is easy to find. Sweep into your socket line, taking care not to join the outer corner to the upper lash line.
- Apply a soft, smudgy line of liner on the upper lash line.
- Apply plenty of mascara, waiting a minute or two between coats so it doesn't get dotted onto your brow bone , as happens so often with hooded eyes.
- Apply a dark tightline under the upper lashes. While this application technique looks great on any eye shape, it's particularly amazing on hooded eyes.
- Lots and lots of mascara will open the eyes a ton.

Prominent

Using the same application technique as round eyes, prominent lids look best if colors are not too light or reflective as they draw too much light to them and can create that "bug eye" look. There's so much lid space on prominent eyes that there's plenty of room for a wide line of liner, smudged out softly, of course.

Now that you know what you are doing, you can move on to the fun stuff, like picking out your colors!!

Eye Popping . . .

Of course, what we all want to achieve is an eye makeup application that makes our eyes "pop"—accentuating our eye color to the fullest. So now, I am going to break down the simplest, most flattering pigments to wear to enhance your eye color.

Bear in mind that there are literally hundreds of thousands of eye shadow colors out there, and narrowing it down to just a few options is no simple task. But since Lazy Perfection makeup errs on the side of natural or natural plus in style and generally doesn't veer into color, trend, or überglammy territory, the colors I am recommending here are the ones that I believe are easiest to apply and the most versatile to wear. You're not going to get a lot of recommendations for red eye shadow or teal eyeliner from me, I'm afraid, and I doubt very much that TPW would ever wear a shadow that's trendy or bright. That's not her style.

BLUE

Use soft, sheer colors with orange or gray undertones like champagne, peach, taupe, soft copper, soft bronze, soft brown, soft gray, and soft navy.

Avoid dense, dark colors like black or purple, which can look too harsh or bruised on blue eyes. Anything that's too pink can make blue eyes look irritated.

GREEN

Use colors with a small amount of pink or red undertones. Champagne pink, peachy pink, beige pink, soft burgundy, soft plum, warm browns, and coppery browns are particularly lovely. Taupe, gray, and dark green in small amounts is also incredibly flattering on green eyes and are some of my personal favorites.

Avoid very bright or icy purples, as they tend to look loud and overdone. Stick to muted violets and plums.

BLUE/GRAY OR GREEN/GRAY

Use all the same colors you would for blue eyes or green eyes, or use any gray-scale colors like taupe, olive, khaki, gunmetal, and charcoal to give a subtle smokiness to the color.

Avoid colors that are very bright; these will distract from the smoky tonality of gray eyes, and anything with too much pink or orange will make them look like you're having an allergy attack.

HAZEL

Use warm, fall tones—gold, rose gold, champagne gold, khaki, olive, evergreen, burgundy, bronze, rich browns, and eggplant. Hazel girls are lucky because you can play up the green or the brown flecks in your eyes and get a different look each time.

Avoid silver and other frosted tones.

BROWN

Use colors that contrast the dark tone of your eyes, either by being lighter or brighter. If your eyes and your eye shadow are too similar in color, it won't have any impact. Stick to warm tonalities like champagne, soft gold, rose gold, deep browns, deep coppers and deep bronzes, and ebony and shades of black.

Avoid colors that have too much white or gray in them, as they can make your eyes look dull and your complexion look ashy.

When selecting your liner, look for the contrast colors in your eyes. If you have flecks of gold or green, rust or amber, blue or grey, that color liner will really make your eyes light up. Black and brown aren't your only options.

> JUST STOP living with pink rims. A few anti redness eye drops will help greatly, as will a soft beige liner in your waterline. Avoid pink or peach liners as they will mix with your redness and make it look worse, and white liner can look too stark. Warm, beige liners will neutralize and counterbalance redness.

Eyes on the Prize

Armed with all the information you need to make some good Lazy Perfection choices, it's time for you to get out the door.

Simple

For running around with the kids; a no-one-to-impress day; going to the gym; getting coffee with a friend; or if you've never worn eye makeup before and want to tiptoe into it.

- Sweep a shadow onto your lid (optional—bare lids are totally fine).
- Tightline under your upper lashes with a deep brown, gray, or soft black.

—AND/OR—

- Smudge a thin line of powder or gel liner along the upper lash line and smudge to soften.
- Add one coat of mascara.

Sophisticated

You have a lunch date, are going to the office, or interviewing for a job; you want to look a little put together but not overdone; or you just want to liven up your makeup look.

- Use eye shadow primer (optional).
- Apply a matte or satin shadow to your lid.
- Apply a deeper matte shadow to your socket line.
- Highlight the inner corner of the eye, the center of the lid, and under the arch of the brow (optional).
- Apply and smudge your liner on your upper and lower lash line.

—OR—

- Tightline.

- Apply one to two coats of mascara.

Sexy

It's date night! Or maybe you're going to a party or an event, or out with a group of friends. This is a longer-wear application technique that will take you from natural to natural plus, with a side of glamour thrown in.

- Apply eye shadow primer.
- Apply a satin finish shadow to your lid.
- Apply a deeper shadow to your socket line and then add an even deeper-toned matte or satin shadow to your outer corner. BLEND.
- Apply pencil liner or gel liner along the upper lash line, smudge to soften, and then add a complementary powder liner on top, also softly smudged, to thicken, soften, and add wear time.
- Apply a powder liner under your lower lash line with or without a touch of pencil liner at the roots of the lashes.
- Tightline (optional).
- Highlight the inner corner of the eye, the center of the base lid, and under the arch of the brow (optional).
- Add two to three coats of mascara on your upper lash line and one to two on your lower lash line.

Eye Candy

No matter your eye color and shape, what makes them look the most beautiful is that they are the windows to your soul. Don't know about you, but when there's the added bonus of gorgeous window treatments and a fabulous view, I'm drawn over to those windows even faster. So get out there and bat those babies!

CHAPTER SEVEN

The Royal We

YOUR EYEBROWS ARE THE ROYALTY OF YOUR FACE. POSITIONED
regally at the very top of your features, they can bestow upon us the
appearance of larger eyes and a more lifted face, not to mention a youthful
countenance. But as brows giveth, so may they taketh away—and the
royal we are certainly not amused by bushy, sparse, or unkempt brows.

All joking aside, the brows, as the tops of your face, can make or break
the rest of your look. Your eye shadow can be beautifully applied, but if
your brows are overgrown or straggly, they can distort the shape of your
eyes, and a queen would never walk among her people looking thus.

Hereditary Rule

While TPW may have been born with brows that are of esteemed lineage,
many of us were not so genetically blessed. I have always envied women
who have thick, dark brows, but I am sorry to say that I am not one
of them. I try, but somehow, filling them in thick and dark looks out
of balance on me. I have learned through personal effort and working
with my clients that even though full brows are in fashion, they always
need to reflect your natural shape, work in concert with your hair color,
personal style and lifestyle, and, of course, your technical skill set. When
considering what the best Lazy Perfection brow approach will be for
you—Simple, Sophisticated, or Sexy—I urge you to keep that in mind.

Ladies in Waiting

It is imperative that your eyebrows live as dutiful, courteous, and upstanding members of the royal court. The way I see it, brows can bring down the entire beauty kingdom should they break with Lazy Perfection protocol and bow when they ought to curtsey. If they're overgrown, or patchy, or so faded and light that you can hardly see them, well, it'd be a shame to let one bad beauty misstep ruin everything. Ladies, I cannot stress enough how important it is to get your brows in good shape.

A Battle Royale

My brows were certainly thicker when I was younger, and most women do experience thinning over time—and the trend toward skinny brows in the 1990s for sure didn't help. The reality is that I *like* to pluck, and the many years of doing so have taken their toll.

JUST STOP looking at your brows in a magnifying mirror. What you see in ten-times enlargement is way more than anyone looking at you would ever notice. If you pluck, do it in a regular mirror with as much light as you can get.

The Royal Treatment

What I recommend to my clients, and what I recommend to you, is getting your eyebrows professionally shaped at least once or twice a year. Believe me, it's an investment worth making, because a professional brow guru can help develop a strategy to get you on track for the most flattering brow shape for you.

A professional can:

- Pluck—done with very sharp tweezers so that hair follicles don't break when they are removed, which can lead to ingrown hairs.
- Thread—done with string to quickly pull away brow hairs—best suited to women with thick, coarse brow hairs.

or

- Wax—done with warm or cold wax that adheres to both the thick and the baby fine hairs and can be sculpted into a very precise shape.

> JUST STOP waxing if you use Retinol. Because of its exfoliating properties, Retinol can thin the skin around the brows, leaving it susceptible to tearing during wax removal.

None of these techniques is for the faint of heart—they all have some degree of discomfort, but when done well, plucking, threading, and waxing all pull the hair follicle out intact, which can extend the amount of time you can go between appointments.

Other advice I strongly suggest you heed is to find a brow specialist on recommendation. Stop someone on the street who has lovely brows and ask her where she goes or check with your most glamorous friend—or even TPW (her brows are great, right?). Walk-ins off the street to service practitioners you don't know can be risky business, and I sure have heard—and seen—some horror stories.

A Royal Coup

No one *wants* bald brows, but I can't begin to tell you how many women come to me with brows that have been so overplucked, they no longer grow. My own mother completely eradicated hers years ago and has to draw them on every day. While she is highly skilled at doing so, talented even, it would be so much easier (read: lazier) if she could simply fill in instead of having to start from scratch.

The good news is that you can successfully stage a coup by using an eyebrow growth stimulant. There are lots of brow and lash stimulants on the market and they work by controlling the growth and shedding stages of the follicles, keeping them in growth state longer. New follicles emerge more quickly, and old follicles fall out less often, giving the appearance of thicker brows, or lashes. They can also bulk up the bulb of the follicle, which makes the hairs come in a little thicker.

> JUST STOP thinking that brow or lash stimulants are going to grow more hair. The fact of the matter is that you cannot create *new* hair follicles—you will always have the exact same number you were born with.

Position, Power, and Prestige

So, before we talk about the many different makeup products and techniques you can use to fill in, thicken, and shape your brows, we have to talk about where they should best be positioned on your face, relative to the rest of your features, so that they may live a life of power and prestige.

How do you know the ideal brow shape for you and your unique bone structure? Grab a brow pencil and let me draw you a map of the palace.

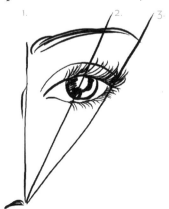

STEP 1—Place the pencil alongside your nose, touching your nostril, and aimed straight up. Make a dot when you get to the point at which your brow bone begins.

STEP 2—Now keep looking straight ahead into the mirror and place the pencil diagonally across the center of your nostril and aim it up toward your brow so that it runs diagonally through your iris, with your pupil as the center point. When you reach the top of your brow, the highest point, make another dot. That's where your arch should be.

STEP 3—Finally, aim the pencil diagonally up from the outer edge of your nostril, lined up with the outer corner of your eye, and up to the tail of your brow. Make a dot—this is where your brow should end.

> **JUST STOP** thinking that there's something drastically wrong if your brows are slightly different shapes, sizes, or thicknesses. Almost everyone has facial asymmetry that can make one look thicker, higher, or longer than the other one, so you should definitely give yourself a break. Your brows are sisters, not twins.

> **JUST STOP** making the tail of your brow too long—this can make your eyes look like they are drooping down at the corners. And also just stop making the tail of your brows too short—this can make your eyes look smaller.

Now, all you have to do is join these three points together to get the ideal shape for you, based on your own anatomy. Believe it or not, there are lots of different ways you can do your brows, and you can do them differently every day. Who'd have thunk that brows could be so versatile—the only thing that should be consistent is the basic three points we just mapped out. Beyond that, I'll show you how they can be filled in thicker, thinner, lighter, darker, with a higher arch, or straighter so that not only can you make them look more tailored, you can make them look more even. It's actually fun to play around with how these variations look on your face.

Noble Lineage

So now that you have your brows in position, you have the power to control what you want them to look like. You can determine their lineage . . . or at least give them a noble line.

Look closely at your brows (fine, use a magnifying mirror for just this one thing) and you will see that there are rows of individual hairs. They're not even rows, set out like seats in the theater, but you can easily distinguish the bottom row and the row just above it.

The row of hairs across the bottom edge should be even, without any stragglers loitering too close and throwing that line off. Even as a professional makeup artist, I find that keeping that row of hairs even can be a challenge. One false move, one hair plucked too close to the bottom edge, and all of a sudden you're a bad mother plucker with an uneven line.

My Lazy Perfection trick is to draw your brows into a clean, well-defined line before you pluck away any strays. Go to town—make it a really dark line so you can clearly see the edge, and then only pluck anything that's underneath it.

And another important tip when self-plucking—only pluck one to two hairs at a time before stepping back from the mirror to make sure you are staying in line. More than that and you may find it a challenge to get your other brow identically shaped. If you're not sure about whether to pluck a particular hair, take it gently with the tweezers and move it out of the way, then step back a little to see what the line of your brow would look like if it were gone. A magnifying mirror is fine for being able to see all the little strays, but when you're checking for shape, it's a far better bet to use a regular mirror and a little distance.

Pretender to the Throne

To make your brows look thicker:

- Start sketching in a line (with pencil, powder, or gel—read on to find out more about them and how they differ) at the very top edge of the brow, slightly higher than the roots of the highest follicles, starting about halfway across the brow, and then complete the line all the way down the top edge of the tail.

- Then, sketch a line on the bottom edge of the brow, starting at the inner corner, moving across until it's lined up directly underneath where the top line starts before angling the pencil (or gel or powder) to the bottom edge of the tail. At this point, you have basically outlined all but the inner/upper line of your brow.

- Start to color in the outline, using short, soft strokes, avoiding the inner corner for now.

- Once the rest of the brow has taken shape and all gaps are colored in, then go back and lightly fill in the inner corner.

JUST STOP creating a heavy, square shape at the inner corner of your brow unless that's what you naturally have. Too much darkness and density in the inner corner can make the eyes look heavy and puffy.

To make the brow look thinner, sketch the outline with concealer instead of a dark brow product, slightly on top of the bottom row of follicles and slightly below the roots of the top follicles, and then repeat the steps as noted above. The concealer will blend into your skin and cover the hairs, creating the illusion of thinner brows.

JUST STOP cutting long brow hairs so short that they have a hard or stubbly-looking edge. Hairs that are a little longer and that can be combed into place look softer and more feminine. If you're worried about long hairs moving out of place over the course of the day, you can set them with some balm or gel.

Color Coronation

When it comes to determining the most flattering color for your brows, there are a couple of fairly simple rules of thumb for keeping them looking natural, and you only need to look as far as your head to figure them out.

- If you have never colored your hair, select a shade of brow product that most closely resembles your natural brow color.
- Light and medium blondes should look for pale, golden, or ashy colors similar to the color of their roots.
- Strawberry blondes and light redheads should match their brows to the tips of their hair. Most redheads have brows that are lighter in color than the hair that grows at the crown of the head, so darkening the brows too much would totally alter their appearance.
- Light and medium brunettes and medium redheads should match their brows to the lightest pieces of their hair. Dark brows and dark hair can be a very beautiful, strong look, but a slightly lighter color brow is softer.
- Dark brunettes and women with black hair should match their hair and their brows almost exactly. This gives a symmetry to the features and a uniformity to the look.
- And women with platinum or gray hair should look for taupe colors, a blend of brown and gray. One exception is if your brows were thick and dark when you were a child, in which case you should attempt to replicate that color.

But as I said earlier, there are a lot of ways to vary your brow look. For daytime, you can keep them lighter in color and thickness and for night you can play them up with slightly darker shades and thicker shapes. For me, as my highlights grow out over the course of several weeks, I deepen the color of my brows to correspond to my roots.

JUST STOP using brow colors that are rusty, coppery, or chestnut unless you are a redhead. If you don't want to look like you just came out of a sauna or as though you had your brows waxed five minutes before, taupe or neutral brown colors are more flattering on most people.

Coronation

Because your brows are the crowning feature of your face, it's okay to help nature along a bit. Filling in your brows to make them look thicker or to adjust their color can be accomplished lots of different ways. Here are brow products that can be used in your coronation.

- **Tinted brow gels or pomades** that look like mascaras are great for filling in already thick brows by coating the hairs with a small amount of pigment, including the odd gray hair. They are also very helpful for anyone who has unruly brows that need to be kept in place. They are not ideal if you need to create shape, fill in patches, or define your line. Simply brush up and into the brows, taking care to wipe excess product off the applicator before doing so in order to avoid clumps.

- **Brow creams or mousses** come in a pot and need to be applied with a brush. The brush is largely responsible for the way these products end up looking, with a sharper-edged brush giving a sharper line and a softer-tipped brush giving a softer line. Brow creams and mousses do a nice job of covering both the hairs and the skin, creating shape and adding volume.

- **Brow pencils** look just like eyeliner pencils and are generally wax based, which means that they adhere to your skin and not to the brow hairs themselves—it's your body heat that allows them to transfer. Translation—in extreme heat conditions, they may melt and get blotchy on the skin. Eyebrow pencils should be kept sharp and may be drawn on with medium to long strokes to create a defined edge or fill in patchy areas.
- **Fine-tipped brow pencils** are perfect for filling in small gaps or patches and for creating a well-defined edge. They are also wax based, but because the tip is much smaller than a regular pencil, there's more precision in the application. Just remember, there is a learning curve with any product that requires precision. Be sure to apply fine-tipped pencils with short, flicky strokes instead of long smooth ones. This will help give the appearance of individual brow hairs.
- **Brow Powder**—Brow powders also need to be applied with a brush, but because the powders grip only on the hairs and not on the skin, they are best suited for anyone who already has fairly robust brows that just need a small amount of fill. Really, any matte eye shadow is fine for this purpose, but many brow powders are sold with two shades that can be mixed and matched with an accompanying wax. The wax may be blotted and blended together with the powder, or used instead of a pomade to hold the brows in place.

I know that with just a little practice, you'll get the hang of how to make the most of your brows to frame your eyes and make your whole face look more lifted and lovely. So now it's time to select the Lazy Perfection Eyebrow Track that's best for you.

Simple

For running out the door, going to meet friends for coffee, going to lunch, or an early morning PTO meeting.

- If your brows are already in pretty good shape, a sweep of clear or tinted brow gel is a fast and easy way to add a small amount of definition and color. If they're a little patchy or out of line, you can dip a brow bush into the gel (or a separate cream or mousse) and apply it directly onto your brow to fill in any sparse areas.

Sophisticated

For lunches out, a meeting in weird, fluorescent office lighting, a casual date night, or when you just need to feel a little more put together.

- Use brow cream, powder, or pencil to fill in patchy areas and give a little definition to your shape without looking like you've spent any time on them.

Sexy

For parties and events, dinners out, special office occasions, or when you're having your headshot done.

- Refine, clean, and shape the edge of your brows with a fine-tipped pencil and then fill in any patchy areas with that same pencil or powder. For extra oomph, set with a small amount of brow gel, making sure to get enough color on the outer tail since that's the part that tends to disappear in photos.

CHAPTER EIGHT

Lip Service

THERE'S A REASON THAT LIPSTICK SALES ARE CONSISTENTLY stronger than any other beauty category out there. It's not just lip service to say that lipstick has an instant and positive impact on us as women—it's a legitimate mood booster. Lonely, frustrated, depressed, or even just bored? Picking up a new lipstick is fun! There's something called "the lipstick effect," which is when lipstick sales go up during tough times—it's instant gratification for a relatively small investment, and it makes us feel confident, optimistic, and excited . . . even if we wake up the next day with buyer's remorse.

Stiff Upper Lip

In truth, though, more than any product, lipstick is the one that seems to have the least amount of buyer's remorse. We just can't seem to keep a stiff upper lip when it comes making an impulse purchase, and so our collections grow and grow and grow. Cheap ones, expensive ones, glossy ones, creamy ones . . . our access to lip products is extensive, which is why I routinely see women in my studio with dozens, and occasionally HUNDREDS of lipsticks in their kits.

In a Lip Lock

This may sound familiar to you. Let's say you're all excited about a special event like a gala or a fund-raiser, and you go get your makeup done so you look sexier and more glam than usual. "You should really go bold with your lip color," the makeup artist says. "It's a great way to dress up your look." Uh-oh . . .

This is a situation that I call the Lazy Perfection Lip Lock. You're not so sure about that lip color, but the makeup artist is veerry persuasive, and you feel like you should trust her because, after all, she's the professional. You feel locked into making that purchase.

Women commonly feel that dressing up their lips dresses up their whole look—and that you need a bold, dramatic color to do it. But in my experience, those are the first lipsticks to go when you do your Lazy Perfection Purge. The ones you get talked into aren't the ones you'll go back to.

It for sure can be fun to play with color, and if you embrace bright colors, then by all means pick yourself up some new ones. But if your basic lipstick choice is ChapStick, it's a big, long leap from there to bright red, dark red, or hot pink. My point is, have some fun and try something new, but just make sure you are going to feel like yourself when you do it. Stepping too far away from your comfort zone can backfire, and you know how important it is to feel confident about your appearance.

JUST STOP allowing yourself to be talked into a new lipstick color by a sales associate. If you are looking to make a change and want to stretch into new territory, it's one thing, but if you have to be talked into it and then only reluctantly agree, you need to listen to your instinct. It's okay to say no. Remember, a good makeup artist won't have ego in her work—she'll just want you to walk away feeling confident and great.

Lip Sync

Lazy Perfection Ladies, I know you want a lip product that you can apply without having to look in the mirror, that you don't have to worry about smudging or taking up residence on your teeth, or that doesn't constantly have to be reapplied. Dramatic lipstick is needy because it requires so much attention, but then, nude lipstick is needy, too, because it requires other makeup to make it look better. Follow along for my Lazy Perfection tips on how to select the one that's juuuust right and totally in (lip) sync with your coloring, lifestyle, and personal style.

You Gotta Kiss a Lot of Frogs

It doesn't make you a lipstick tramp to get out there and kiss a whole lot of frogs in pursuit of your lipstick Prince Charming. Not to worry, there will be no lip shaming in this book because some of those frogs are pretty decent kissers, if you know what I mean. You should enjoy playing the frog field—there's no reason to make a big investment or commit to just one color. There's more than one perfect lip product for you—you just need to know what you like and what you don't. So to help you start your reptilian romance off right, here are the different lip formulations—textures—from which you can choose, from the lightest and most sheer to the most opaque and dense.

- Tinted lip balms—With or without SPF protection, lip balms are generally sheer in color and feel hydrating on the lips. Anyone can wear them, and they are easy to apply.
- Lip gloss—Lip gloss is generally a sheer, thin texture, with or without shimmer, that adds shine to lips. Lip gloss can be applied alone or on top of other lip products, and can also be mixed and matched together.

I generally do not advocate mixing glosses together as it seems to defeat the Lazy Perfection purpose. There are thousands of lip gloss options out there—surely you can find one that works without needing to be mixed.

- **Lip stains**—Generally a sheer, liquidy formulation, stains serve as a long-wear base to other lip colors and remain present when those partner lip products wear away. May be drying on the lips.

- **Satin lipstick**—This is the most flattering, forgiving formula for most women. It has a slight sheen to it but still packs a demi-opaque punch of color. A small amount of shine on the lips gives them the appearance of being fuller and more hydrated.

- **Chubby lip pencils**—Available in a wide range of colors and textures, chubby lip pencils are a hybrid of a lipstick and a lip pencil, hugging the curves of the lips for a slightly more defined application. Some need to be sharpened and others do not, but they are generally convenient to carry and apply.

- **Cream lipstick**—Slightly less shine and slightly more color than a satin lipstick, cream formulations bring a little more depth and opacity to the lips.

- **Demi-/semi-matte lipstick**—The love child of matte and satin lipsticks. Can be worn by anyone more comfortably than matte.

- **Matte lipstick**—Totally free from sheen, shimmer or shine, matte lipsticks can be flattering on young, smooth lips, but on older ones, may accentuate fine lines, look dry and/or dull, and give the impression that the lips are thin.

- **Long-wear lipstick**—Long-wear lipsticks are often densely packed with pigments and are full-coverage in terms of color payoff. They may be housed in a traditional lipstick, in a gel formulation, or as a liquid that dries and sets in place. They may be worn with or without gloss on top and are well suited for long days or special events as they do not need frequent reapplication. Like matte lipsticks and stains, they can be drying.

And then there's:

• Lip liner—Lip liner comes in pencil form and is used to define and shape the outline of the lips. Most flattering and versatile in a shade that matches your natural lip color, when used strategically, lip pencils can also improve the appearance of volume and plumpness. When used in a color that is too dark or too bright, or drawn on in a heavy manner, lip pencils look dated and obvious.

Bad-Mouthing

So, lip-plumping products are a bit controversial. Some women swear by them while others see little to no results at all. They are generally formulated with irritants, such as mint, peppers, or cinnamon that cause increased swelling and circulation in the lips, and a glossy finish that gives the illusion of a fuller pout. If you're okay with a tingling or burning sensation on the lips, then go for it. But if your lips are dry, or prone to dryness, approach with caution as they can perpetuate a dry skin cycle. And while we're at it . . .

JUST STOP using "moisturizing" ChapSticks or lip balms that contain menthol or camphor. They feel great when you first put them on, but then end up sucking all the moisture out of your lips, making you think you need to apply more. That's why people describe them as addictive.

True Love's Kiss

Don't be a hero. You cannot depend on your lipsticks or lip glosses alone to provide you with adequate moisture for your lips. Sometimes you need true love's kiss to bring you back from the brink.

Because the skin on our lips is so thin and delicate, and because there are no oil glands in them, they are particularly prone to dryness and chapping. The only effective way to keep them hydrated is to drink plenty of water so you don't get dehydrated or develop dry mouth, and use an occlusive balm, meaning something that holds in what little moisture they have and protects them against the elements like sun, wind, and cold. Products like coconut oil, Vaseline and Aquaphor are ideally applied a few times a day, but at the very least, when you go to sleep or when you are flying. Waxy lip balms can also help hold in moisture, but additional ingredients in them such as fragrance or flavor can negate all the hydrating benefits. And finally, if you use AHAs or BHAs when you wash your face, put a little balm on before so that they won't get direct access to the lips and cause irritation.

On Everyone's Lips

Lip product selection is a highly individual choice, but everyone should have at least four different lipstick textures that can be used separately or in combination—whatever fits your whim. Here are my Lazy Perfection product selections that I think should be on everyone's lips.

• Lip balm

• Satin lipstick

• Chubby lip pencil OR demi-matte lipstick OR cream lipstick

• Lip Gloss

While it's not the *laziest* of Lazy Perfection, all these textures work in sync, can easily be layered and mixed, so you'll always have new ways to keep your look fresh and interesting.

Put Your Money Where Your Mouth Is

The vast majority of my clients come to me with a minimum of six lip products—and sometimes as many as two hundred—many of which are basically the same color. I get it—once we find an easy, natural-looking color, we want to stick with it, but there's enough variation from brand to brand, and product to product, that the difference between pale rose and light rose feels like a whole new direction, so we plunk down our money and put it right back onto our lips. After all, we love rose! Far be it from me to suggest that you stop buying so many lipsticks. It can, after all provide instant gratification and an ego boost. However, in general terms, I maintain that for true Lazy Perfection, keeping just four colors in your kit will give you enough variety to keep things interesting. Here is what I suggest:

1) LIPS AU NATUREL

It's all about the nudes and how you can rock them to feel your sexiest. They are not easy to choose, to be honest. There are more nudes than there are dimples in my thighs, but with these Lazy Perfection tips, I can help smooth the way to choosing the one that's right for you.

The best nudes are just a hair darker or a hair lighter than your natural lip color. And by a hair, I mean, a tiny bit. Big shade variance will defeat the purpose—if it's much darker, it's just another lipstick, and if it's too much lighter, you'll look like the walking dead. Super not cute.

JUST STOP thinking that nude lipsticks should be the same shade as your skin. If your face is monochromatic, you'll look washed out and oxygen deprived.

When determining your best nude, stand slightly back from the mirror a bit and assess whether your lips are naturally pale—are the edges are similar in color to the skin around them, or naturally pigmented, or do they stand out against your skin? This will be your baseline for selecting a light nude or a darker nude. The basic nude colors are:

Beige nude—Great for pale lips and fair to light complexions.

Pink nude—Works for pale or rosy lips in fair to medium complexions. As with all pinks, there are millions of shades that can be milky, rosy, mauve, or berry in color.

Peachy nude—Good for pale lips but will clash with naturally rosy or brown lips. Works for fair to medium complexions. They can be peachy/pink or more orange in color.

Caramel nude—Works for brown pigmented lips and comes in a range of shades from light to dark. Lovely for medium/dark to dark complexions.

Brown nude—Works for dark pigmented lips on medium/dark to dark complexions.

One of the best things you can do when trying to find your nudity is to take twenty dollars with you to a big box or drugstore and buy as many different options as you can, then try them all before making a bigger investment in a designer product. This way, you'll get a sense of the nude color that's the most flattering before you decide whether you want or need to spend more on a luxury formulation. But hey—if you like one that you found at a drugstore, there's no reason you have to switch away from it.

> JUST STOP thinking that designer lipsticks or glosses are "better" than drugstore ones. The fact of the matter is, they all need to be reapplied with some frequency, so it really doesn't matter if you spend five dollars or forty-five dollars. If you prefer the feel, fragrance, or packaging of a designer product, well that's a different story.

And if you haven't had any success with choosing the right nude, you can stop beating yourself up, because sometimes it's not the lipsticks' fault. There are some basic things you should be doing with your other makeup in order to balance and enhance the look of nude lips.

- With a pale nude, such as pink or peach, use a light wash of blush in the same color family.
- Add more definition around the eyes and brows to give more strength to the features on the upper part of the face. Extra or slightly darker eyeliner, another coat of mascara, and a well-shaped brow will make a huge difference.
- Make sure that all discoloration in your skin has been neutralized with concealer and/or foundation. Skin that's blotchy will make a nude lip look washed out.
- With darker nudes or darker skin tones, make sure you add some contrast to the complexion and eyes, such as a gold or peachy gold bronzer or highlighter or shadow to attract light and add glow.

2) PUCKER UP PEACH

Warm colors, those with a little hint of peach in them, are flattering on pretty much everyone. The key is to select a peach that works with your natural lip color. If you have deep, brown lips, then a stronger peach/ orange, will be most flattering. Conversely, if you have pale lips, a light, milky peach will look best. Your peachy lip color and your peachy blush color should live on the same block. They might not be next-door neighbors, but they should at least carpool to work together.

3) ROSE LIPS SINK SHIPS

Pale rose, dusty rose, peachy rose, baby rose, hot rose . . . there is a pink-toned lip color that will suit everyone, and bonus . . . rose lipsticks can be dabbed and blended on the cheeks to perk up the complexion as well. Pink tones give a youthful poutiness to the lips and make them look fresh and healthy.

Do me a favor, and suspend your vanity for a moment. We're going to do a little exercise to help determine your best rose. Look in a mirror and pull your lower lip out and down. Feeling silly yet? Just hang on . . . There's a lot of blood flow in the mouth, so the color you see on your inner lower lips is a pretty good indicator of which tone of pink will be most flattering for you. Choose one that's one to two shades darker or one to two shades lighter than this. I have been caught many times in beauty departments pulling my lip out in order to assess my best color . . . The things we do in the name of beauty, eh?

4) BERRY BIG MOUTH

And finally, there is a shade of berry that will add drama and edge to your look, whether you like it sheer, opaque, or matte. Berry colors typically are a blend of pink, blue, and brown, so the range is extensive, from plum to fuchsia and anything in between. A word to the wise—very dark colors on thin lips will make them look thinner. If you want to wear a deep, dramatic color but your lips lack any degree of trout-pout, then a touch of lip liner to frame the shape with a dab of gloss on top will attract the light and give the impression of more plumpness.

Red My Lips

Oh my goodness. If I had a nickel for every time I heard or read that there's a red lipstick for everyone, I'd be super wealthy. Sure, with enough effort, I'm sure everyone could probably could find a flattering red, but red lipstick is about way more than just the color. Red lipstick is a bold, attention-grabbing, style-defining "look," and not necessarily suitable for everyone. In Lazy Perfection Land, red lipstick needs to work in concert with everything else in your look. Red requires a little more effort to apply evenly—one false swipe and you look smudgy instead of chic—and it also requires the right attitude.

We've been told that a sweep of red lipstick is all the makeup you need, but sometimes that just looks crazy instead of chic. If you have blotchy skin, patchy brows, or dark circles, and then you apply nothing but a red lipstick, well that can backfire faster than a classic coupe. And let me assure you—you probably already know this one—it won't necessarily make you feel like a walking, talking sexified powerhouse. Personally, I think that red requires too much effort, and I am just far too lazy for it.

If you feel the same as I do, when you're getting ready for a glam event, you can try a nude color with a darker eye for that Victoria's Secret sexy-girl-next-door look, or a warm rosy color with a sheer gloss on top for Julia Roberts–level glamour, or a coppery peach à la Julianne Moore. There's more to getting glam than just a red lip. You can be confident, empowered, sexy, and strong in ANY lip color that makes you feel fabulous.

Smart Mouth

Lazy Perfection is all about education, and learning to identify what you like and what you don't. You got a whole mouthful (from me) about the Lazy Perfection lip look, and now it's up to you to decide how you're going to sync those lips.

Simple

This is for anyone who just wants a no-brainer throw-on.

- A sweep of nude balm, gloss, or satin lipstick adds the appearance of hydration to the lips and draws the light to them, which in turn perks up the complexion.

Sophisticated

If you want to add just a little extra something-something to your look, you can layer any of these products together.

- Satin lipstick or a chubby pencil in nude, rose, peach, or berry give a little more shape and depth to the lips and a hint more color to the face. These are both daytime- and evening-appropriate and can be reapplied without having to look in a mirror.

Sexy

This is for maximum va-voom, when you know you need long-wear or a little extra drama, like at a black tie event, a special dinner, or when you're going to your high school reunion and know for sure that TPW is going to be there.

- For a more defined and fuller-looking lip, subtly line with a lip-colored pencil, making sure to sketch the line and smudge it together, as a solid line looks too obvious. Layering a richly pigmented lipstick, like a demi-matte or cream, with a touch of gloss on top increases the depth of the color and the drama. If you want to avoid having to reapply with frequency, a stain or long-wear can be added as the first step.

The Lazy Perfection Lip Synch will help you buy the lipstick that you know is going to make you look and feel great. Let's dub it the Lazy Perfection effect.

CHAPTER NINE

Isn't It Romantic?

I HAVE TO PUT IT OUT THERE—THERE'S A REASON THAT ONE OF the hottest-selling blushes of all time was given the racy name "Orgasm." I try to avoid using this particular blush when I'm working with younger teens or teen models—I just don't want to open the door to that conversation (yikes)—but the fact of the matter is that love, sex, and romance do leave a lovely flush on the cheeks, the kind that looks natural and fresh (if not innocent). Who knows what goes on behind closed doors, but TPW for sure has the kind of radiant, rosy skin that doesn't need a lot of blush. Maybe she has a life filled with romance, or maybe she just never leaves home without putting on blush. For most of us, a dash of color on the cheeks is the number one way to give our complexions a pop of passion.

At First Blush

I can't tell you how many times people have said to me, "If I knew I was going to see you, I would have put on more makeup." It always strikes me as funny, because when I talk to someone, I barely even notice their makeup. I always tell them, "I am talking to YOU, not your makeup." I suppose they are scared that because I am a professional makeup artist I am constantly evaluating their makeup.

Truthfully, the only time I notice someone's makeup is when it's overapplied or underblended, and honestly, unblended blush is one of the most common makeup faux pas I see. But I don't judge, because I know that the problem is likely one of three things. She's either using a formula or color that is incompatible with her foundation or skin type; she doesn't understand her facial anatomy; or her makeup brush isn't in tip-top condition. All three missteps are very easy to correct, and it is my pleasure to help you learn how.

Made for Each Other

I love a good cheek, one with a natural-looking flush and a radiant glow, the kind that you get when you are in the early stages of a new romance. One of the most consistent features in my work as a makeup artist is a strong cheek—I just love the way it livens up the face. That doesn't necessarily mean that the color of the blush has to be bright or dark, more that the cheek brings the overall look of vibrancy to the face, the way a good accessory can perk up your outfit. An underdone cheek can wash out your whole look, so even if you've applied beautiful shadow or lips, you can end up looking dull and flat. There are so many different blush formulas out there, so let me walk you through what they are and whether you and your blush are made for each other.

- Powder—This is the most commonly used type of blush and comes in matte, satin (light shimmer), or full-shimmer finishes. Powder blushes work best for normal, combination, oily, and acne-prone skin but aren't super friendly to dry skin as they can accentuate flaws or float on top of the pores. Powder blushes are best applied on top of other powders, such as setting or bronzer, so that it won't grip into any residual cream or oil left on your skin. Mismatched texture is the number one cause of blush blotchiness.

JUST STOP thinking that you need to press down hard on your brush when you are applying blush. If the bristles on your brush are indented or crushed in the center, you are pressing too hard, which makes it more difficult to get a smooth application. Blush should be softly applied and built up in light layers until you reach your desired level of color. Remember, it's easier to add color than it is to take away.

- **Cream**—Somewhere along the way, cream blush became the wicked stepmother of the makeup world, but it seems to be having a bit of a renaissance. Cream blush is most often sheer to light in coverage and gives a natural, subtle glow since it melds so well with the natural texture of skin (no one has naturally powdery skin, right?) It comes in matte and shimmer, and can be housed in pans, sticks, or tubes. Cream blush is great for normal and dry complexions but may have less wear time on oily or combination skin, unless it's layered under a corresponding powder blush to give extra grip. Also, if you are prone to breakouts, the emollient ingredients in cream blush may clog your pores. It can be applied with fingers or a brush in a swirling, sweeping, or tapping motion, but the most important thing with cream blush is to ensure that the edges of the application are blended away so that they don't look obvious.

- **Liquid blush and serum blush**—Liquids and serums are thin and watery in consistency. Because of their thin texture, they apply well with a brush or a sponge, but fingers definitely aren't the way to go here as they can cause streaking. Serum blushes often have the added benefits of skincare ingredients and are most compatible with normal or dry skin, but if it comes in a long-wear, aka "stain" formulation, it may be equally suitable for oily or combination skin.

- **Stain**—Cheek stains are very watery in consistency, strong on pigmentation, and set to a long-wear finish very, very quickly. Like, lickety-split. Like, if you don't blend it right away, you will look like you have broken out in a weird rash. It's best to apply with fingers so that you can work it into place as quickly as possible, but if you are left with a blotch or an edge, buffing with a damp sponge will help to smooth it out. Stains are less than ideal for dry skin or applied over powder as they can grab on to flaky patches and look splotchy. For smooth, oily, or combination skin, stains work very well.

- **Gel**—Gel blushes are relatively new and are a hybrid between cream and stain. They apply like a cream, becoming one with the skin (super Zen) but then set in place like a stain. They can also be applied with fingers, but a damp sponge or a brush will ensure a smoother blend. This is a great option for oily skin, but gel blushes will work on all skin types.
- **Cream to Powder**—Just as it sounds, it applies like a cream but wears like a powder. Great for any skin type, but especially oily or combination.

So just to sum up, here's a little chart showing you what type of blush is best for you, based on your skin type.

SKIN TYPE	POWDER	CREAM	LIQUID/ SERUM	GEL	CREAM TO POWDER	STAIN
Normal	X	X	X	X	X	X
Oily	X			X	X	X
Dry		X	X	X		
Combination	X			X	X	X

Liaison Location

This is important. Almost as important as selecting the type and color of your blush. Where you place it on your cheeks, the liaison location, is CRUCIAL in getting a natural look. Here is a little chart of the anatomy of a cheek.

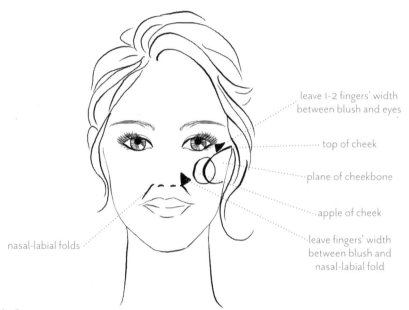

leave 1-2 fingers' width between blush and eyes

top of cheek

plane of cheekbone

apple of cheek

leave fingers' width between blush and nasal-labial fold

nasal-labial folds

Let's dissect.

- Blush should be placed in the horizontal center of the face, no higher than one to two fingers' width from your lower lash line and no lower than the tip of the nose.

    Blush that's placed too high on the face looks unnatural and can make it look long.

    Blush that's too low makes the cheeks look flattened out and droopy.

- There should be one to two fingers' widths between your blush and your nostrils.

If your blush is too close to the nose it can accentuate redness and make you look like you have a bad cold, or call attention to the nasal-labial folds (most unappealing name for a facial feature ever.).

- There should be one to two fingers' width between the top of your blush and the outer corners of your eyes.

  Blush that's too close to the eyes can accentuate fine lines and wrinkles.
- The apples of your cheeks start higher than you think they do. Try this:

  1) Make an O shape with your index finger and thumb, covering your index finger nail completely with your thumb.

  2) Now smile, and place the O onto the apples of your cheeks making sure that the entire O sits flush to the skin and that the fleshiest part is what's peeking through the middle.

  3) Your thumbnail should be pointing up, and the bend in the knuckle should lightly rest against the side of your nostril.

  4) With your other index finger, point right into the center of the O. That's where you want to aim your blush, blending outward from there. If you place your blush too low on the apple of your cheek, when you stop smiling, the blush placement will flatten out the appearance of your cheeks. Droopy Dog central.

The Perfect Couple

Your blush brush needs to be your best friend so it's one of the tools in your kit worth investing in—you simply cannot be the perfect couple without it. I'm not going to brush-shame any of my clients, but plenty of them have come to me over the years with brushes so dried out, dented, broken, and shedding that the shape is no longer distinguishable. It makes perfect sense that there's simply no way to get a smooth application of blush if your brush is in bad condition.

JUST STOP thinking that you don't have to bother taking care of your brushes. If you don't wash them at least once a month (or once a week if your skin is very oily or prone to breakouts), not only will oils build up on the bristles and make them less flexible and less able to pick up product from the pan, but over time, the bristles will begin to dry out and break off. You wouldn't skip washing your hair for months at a time, would you?

You should feel free to use either a synthetic or a natural hair brush—whichever feels best to you—but, generally speaking, liquids and cream apply better with synthetic brushes and powders apply better with natural bristles. The reason . . . natural bristles, like our own hair, absorb a certain amount of the emollients in cream products, so they don't give an even distribution on the skin, whereas synthetic hairs aren't at all porous and can put all the makeup from the bristles directly onto the skin. You with me so far?

There are some natural hair brushes that are dense enough to work with liquids and creams. I carry them in my own line and use them in my kit. And of course there are synthetic brushes that work beautifully with powder. I also have them in my own line and kit. It really just boils down to personal preference and budget.

But more important than the synthetic/natural debate is the shape and size of your brush and whether it works in concert with your facial structure. Big, fluffy brushes are so appealing, and we tend to think that they'll get our makeup on faster because they cover more surface area—but when it comes to your cheeks, always remember it's about location, location, location. A brush that's too big is not going to place the product where it should be.

I know that makeup brushes aren't easy for everyone to understand, but I always tell my clients to use common sense and let the shape be your guide. Picasso couldn't paint a straight sharp line with a domed-shaped brush, and he couldn't get a soft, diffused application with a brush that has a sculpted, flat edge.

But in no way do you need to be an artist, makeup or otherwise, to understand blush brushes. Here is all you really need to know:

- A rounded, domed brush will give you a round, soft shape and is perfect for blending into the apples of the cheeks.
- A flattened domed brush (what I call flat/fluffy) will be the most versatile, hugging the planes of the cheekbones but still able to buff into the apples. This shape is the most common for blush brushes.
- An angled brush hugs the bottom of the cheekbone, allowing for a more contoured/sculpted application.
- Densely packed brushes will pick up more product from the pan and drag it onto the skin, which is fine as long as you don't use too much pressure that can overly stretch the skin or distort the shape of your cheek.
- Softer, more flexible brushes will pick up less product from the pan and whisper it onto the skin.
- Soft versus dense is personal preference.

Cheek to Cheek

It's totally worth noting that if you have experienced weight gain or weight loss and the fatty deposits in your cheeks have plumped up or fallen south, blush will be your very best friend. Here are some very simple tricks for creating whatever illusion you need.

If you have gained weight, a sweep upward along the cheekbone with a brown-based color like rose or mocha will sculpt the face and create the impression that the lower part of your face is very slim. Aim your flat/fluffy or angled brush along the lower ridge of your cheekbone, lined up with the corner of your mouth and the center of your ear cartilage.

Conversely, if you have lost weight and your cheeks have fallen a bit or look sunken, a sweep of blush high onto the apples of the cheeks draws attention and light to the plumpest part of the cheek and creates the impression of more roundness. Be careful here, though—if you apply blush too low on the apple, when you stop smiling and your face is at rest, it will give a saggy effect. Do the O-Trick outlined earlier in this chapter, but instead of aiming for the center of the O, aim for the top of the O. Use small, round motions when blending your blush into place, taking care to diffuse the edges so you don't end up looking like you have circles on each cheek.

Making Beautiful Music

There is ZERO doubt in my mind that TPW has never, in her life, had blotchy, splotchy blush. She knows how to work her blend, and always looks like her flush is just radiating from the inside out. She probably also knows the cardinal rule of good blush application: your foundation and blush textures need to work in concert.

- Cream blush and her cousins, Serum, Liquid, Gel, and Stain, are viscous and fluid. Cream foundation is viscous and fluid. Brava—a lovely harmony.
- Powder blush is soft and floaty. Powder foundation is soft and light. A perfect duet.
- Cream blush and all her cousins are viscous and fluid. Powder foundation is soft and light. Wah wah. The cream blush will rub away the powder underneath it.
- Powder blush is soft and floaty; cream foundation is viscous and fluid.... Scrreeeech. It's like nails on a chalkboard. Blotch City.

The only way to ensure that powder blush works in concert with cream foundation is to lightly dust a little setting powder or bronzer onto your cheeks to lay down a barrier layer between them. This will absorb some of the viscosity in your cream foundation and create a compatible texture onto which your powder blush can float. Always remember, your skin and your cheeks must live together in harmony, both in the textural compatibility and the way your blush gets blended on your cheeks.

We have some of the key blush points covered now—what kind is best for your skin; where to apply it; and the tool with which to apply it. Now we get to move on to the fun stuff . . . Choosing your color.

Torn between Two Lovers

I believe that most women, especially the Lazy Perfection Woman, only needs two blushes in her kit. There is a shade of peach and a shade of pink that will work for everyone, so I advise you to steer clear of trendy colors altogether and go with these two classics. Styles may change over the years, as may your preference for cream versus powder, but there is nothing that's ever going to compete with the gorgeous flush of a natural pink or peachy cheek. So—choose peach, pink, or one of each. You don't have to be torn between them.

Peach tones work for EVERYONE. Fair, dark, olive, sallow . . . you name it and there is a shade of peach that will suit your skin. Why? Because the little bit of orange in the mixture warms up the complexion and gives a lovely, subtle glow.

And there is a pink for everyone, but to be fair, *pink* and *peach* in Blush World are the same as *beige* in Concealer World. There are millions of variations, no two are alike, and everyone has a slightly different interpretation of what *peach* and *pink* mean.

But the good news is that in Blush World, just like in Concealer World, there are top-selling blush colors in every line because they are the ones that are the most versatile. The makeup associates reach for them over and over again because they work well on so many different people, so you can always just ask for them instead of driving yourself crazy trying to figure it out.

If you feel up to the challenge of figuring it out yourself, I'm going to tell you exactly what colors work best on all the different skin tones but really it comes down to this—light colors for light skin and bright colors for darker skin. If you're somewhere in between—as about 80 percent of women are—your blush should be somewhere in between as well.

Let's do a little review of blush color vocabulary because it can be terribly confusing.

- **Petal pink/baby pink**—A milky, pale pink. Think of baby showers and carnations. Lovely on fair skin.
- **Peach**—Literally, think of the skin of a peach (not the inside). Soft pink/orange/yellow blend. Great for pale and light complexions.
- **Natural pink**—A soft brown-based pink, but not too pink, and not too brown. Super subtle but flattering on light and medium complexions.
- **Peachy pink**—This is a confusing one because there are so many interpretations. Basically, it's like the modern version of coral, only toned down. Any blend of peach and pink, whether they are light or dark. Great for light, medium, and medium-dark complexions.
- **Apricot**—A darker version of peachy pink, heavier on the orange, but still with some pink tonality. Great for medium and medium-dark complexions.
- **Coral**—Any combination of pink and orange, but generally more orange. It's the original peachy pink—just a little louder and brighter. Works for light, medium, and medium-dark complexions, depending on the intensity of the color.
- **Rose**—Falls in the same category as peachy pink, in that it comes in a million variations. Most commonly, rose blush has a warm, almost

brown base and is very flattering on medium complexions. Paler rose colors also suit light tones.

- Mauve—A cool-toned, medium pink. Has some blueness to it. Great for medium and medium-dark complexions.
- Berry—A red-based pink. Wonderful on medium, medium-dark, and dark skin tones.
- Watermelon—A bright, blue-based pink, also wonderful on medium, medium-dark, and dark skin tones.
- Hot pink—See berry and watermelon, only on crack.
- Tangerine—A medium-orange tone that looks beautiful on dark complexions.
- Bronzed pink—Pink with a bronze undertone. Lovely for light and medium complexions.
- Mocha—Any shade of pink with a cool brown undertone. Good for medium and medium-dark complexions.
- Plum—A darker, slightly more purple version of Mocha. Ideal for dark complexions.
- Brick red—A rich, warm red. Suits dark skin.

JUST STOP thinking that the way a blush looks *off* your face is the way it will look on your face. Don't forget that, housed in its container, all the pigments in the blush are compressed, making it look stronger. When the color particles get broken apart and spread around, they become softer and less jarring. Some blushes do have more color payoff than others, so swatching on the back of your hand is a good way to test the strength of the color.

It's Getting Serious

The flush of first love has deepened to something more, so it's time now for you Lazy Perfection girls to decide what is going to give you the fastest, prettiest, most glowing look, and take your relationship with blush to the next, more serious level. Choose your track!

Simple

Stain (for oily skin), powder, or cream, in a sheer formula, blended with fingers or a brush onto the apples of the cheeks. This will give a subtle sheen to the complexion but not look out of place if you have no other makeup on.

Sophisticated

Cream or powder in a matte or satin finish, light to medium coverage, applied with a brush along the underside of the cheekbone and then lightly blended onto the apples. This will give shape and definition to the cheeks, slim the face, and bring brightness to the complexion.

Sexy

For long-wear or to bump up the intensity of your blush look, apply a light wash of cream or gel blush onto the apples of the cheeks and along the cheekbones and then lightly dust a corresponding powder blush color on top, from the same brand or different. If you are going to be wearing black, be in a dark environment, or know that your photo will be taken, add 20 percent more blush than you usually would so that you don't look washed out.

I've always had a blush crush, but so many women have never been able to find Mr. Right Blush. You can call me a Lazy Perfection Matchmaker, because now you have the absolute best way to find the blush of your dreams.

CHAPTER TEN

Lazy Perfection Punctuation

Putting a Period on It

WHO'D HAVE THOUGHT WE'D BE TALKING ABOUT GRAMMAR IN a beauty book, right? But hear me out—punctuation marks can complete your thought, reflect your emotion, and add a layer of dimension that brings nuance and suggestion. And since Lazy Perfection is all about adding small but significant details, punctuation seems like a fitting last step.

There are several makeup products and techniques that, while not absolutely *necessary* to a daily beauty routine, do give extra inflection to your look. The Lazy Perfection Tracks laid out in the previous chapters—Simple, Sophisticated, and Sexy—are all well-rounded and complete, and can end right where they are with a solid and decisive period. But now it's time to decide whether you want to add additional flavor. A suggestive "..." with bronzer perhaps, or an enthusiastic "!" with highlighter, or even a transformational ";" with a lash curler ... These little marks lead the reader (or in the case of makeup, the viewer) to a more fully expressed thought. That's why using small details of makeup punctuates your look.

Footnotes

So, think of your makeup application the same way you would think about writing a term paper. You have to support your themes by giving evidence to shore up your point. The footnotes are the behind-the-scenes effort that can make or break the grade you get. Here are some ways you can prove your beauty thesis even more conclusively.

Bronzer Brackets

I want to go on record here and say that I am a HUGE fan of bronzer. Were it not for the fact that I have worked with thousands of women who have never in their lives considered using it, I would even go as far as saying that it's a Lazy Perfection NECESSITY. But, in deference to our individual needs and styles, I will back off and say instead that it is my most recommended punctuation product.

Bronzer is so misunderstood. Granted, errors in usage are perhaps more frequent and more obvious with bronzer than with any other makeup product. How many times have you seen an orange politician? A reality star with dark lines streaked across her face? A newscaster who looks so deeply sun damaged that it distracts from the news? There's no question that a heavy-handed application of bronzer can destroy an otherwise lovely makeup look, but bronzer can also, when used correctly, be the most forgiving, helpful, flattering makeup product of them all.

JUST STOP thinking that you have to choose either bronzer or blush. They can absolutely be worn separately, but they can also be worn together, as long as you take care to blend them well.

Here are the many ways in which bronzer should be appreciated and embraced.

- It can bridge the color gap between the face, neck, and chest.
- Pale, dull, or tired skin is not youthful or fresh. A light sweep of bronzer can add warmth and vibrancy.
- When gravity takes a toll, bronzer can step in to lift the appearance of jawline, cheeks, and eyelids.
- When suffering from redness, bronzer can neutralize and distract.
- When one product has been overapplied or isn't looking balanced, bronzer is the mediator who negotiates peace. If your eyes look too dark and the rest of your face is washed out, a sweep of bronzer is a fast, easy solution.

JUST STOP using hard, stiff, or oversized brushes to apply your bronzer. They grab too much product from the pan, don't blend easily, and don't give you a lot of control in where it gets applied. For a natural and subtle application of bronzer, it's important to use a very soft, domed-shaped brush that will swirl it lightly onto the most flattering areas of the face, and give an even, smooth blend.

Color Question Mark

What color should my bronzer be? That's the number one question I hear from my clients. Bronzers should be no more than two shades darker than your skin or about the same level of tan you would achieve naturally. Too much darker and you start to get into reality star territory, and, of course, super orange or super red colors are best avoided.

The second-most common question—should it be matte or sparkly? Your bronzer should have little to no shimmer and no visible sparkly particles. Metallic or glitter bronzers do not look natural. If you can, hold up different bronzers from different brands against each other to compare the degree of orange, swatch on the back of your hand to determine whether the glitter particles are going to be too obvious, or research swatches online before you buy.

> **JUST STOP** thinking that there's a one-size-fits-all color for bronzer. Just because a particular brand may be a best-seller does not mean it will be right for you. It means that it was right for the ad campaign. In short, don't believe everything you read, and choose a color that's YOUR best fit.

Edges and Ellipses . . .

Making your bronzer look like naturally sun-kissed skin is all about aiming for the outer edges of your face so that you look glowing and warm, not like you're trying to fake the kind of all-over tan you would get from sitting out on the beach in Hawaii (where you should really be under an umbrella, in a hat, wearing SPF 5000, of course) or in a tanning booth (which, ew—please don't do that. So bad for you!).

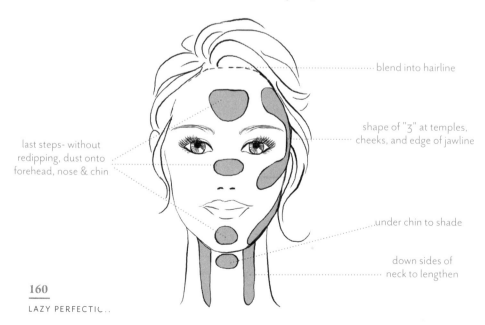

blend into hairline

shape of "3" at temples, cheeks, and edge of jawline

last steps- without redipping, dust onto forehead, nose & chin

under chin to shade

down sides of neck to lengthen

- First and most important—remember to start slowly and add more color as you need it. Lightly dip or swirl the brush into the pan and then TAP OFF THE EXCESS POWDER. You know it's way easier to add more than to take away, and since there is quite a lot of pigment in bronzer and such a high rate of error, this tapping step is essential.
- Start on the cheeks, blending back and forth where you would usually apply blush, aiming just underneath the cheekbone. This is a larger area of the face so there's room to move and blend the product.
- Without redipping, take the brush up onto the temples and across the hairline, sweeping lightly back and forth.
- Sweep back down onto the cheeks and just under the cheekbone, aim back up toward the ear, and then turn the corner down onto the jawline. You're making the shape of the number 3 on the outer edges of your face. If you want even more color, dip your brush again, tap away the excess, and start from the beginning.
- Always check to see if you need bronzer on your neck and décolletage to ensure that they match the color of your face. I personally try to do this step every single day, as my face is naturally darker than my neck and chest.
- Sweep what's left on the brush onto the forehead, nose and chin.

"Bronzer" Versus "Contour"— Quotation Mark Smackdown

You may be wondering, are bronzing and contouring different and do I have to do both? Well, yes and no. Contouring is another Lazy Perfection punctuation step because it's a great way to create and define shape on the face, and it works beautifully when paired with highlighting. For anyone who has gained or lost weight, or who is starting to see gravity take its toll, contouring can hollow out our cheeks, elongate our necks, lift our jawlines, enlarge our eyes, and slim our noses.

But . . . a contour is just a way to create a shadow with makeup, so the color has to be a little on the gray side, as natural shadows are, and the finish should be matte—because shadows don't sparkle. Bronzers are generally more in the golden brown color spectrum and may have a little shimmer.

A professional artist, or anyone who is willing to put in more time than with the Lazy Perfection approach, may want to keep her bronzer and contour products separate. An orange or shimmery product simply won't create the appearance of a natural shadow, and conversely, a gray-based, matte color isn't going to enliven the complexion—it'll just make you look like a vampire.

But . . . there are bronzers that can function both to enliven and freshen up the skin and create natural, convincing shape. Simply put, you need to stay away—far away—from bronzers that are too orange, too gray, or too shimmery. Think of something like the color of a roasted chicken—a warm, baked, brown. And for ladies with a darker complexion, think of a well-done roasted chicken, with a hint of sautéed onion.

I know it can be hard to tell the difference between colors when you are looking at them alone, but as mentioned earlier, if you can hold them up against other bronzers, swatch on the back of your hands, or search swatch images online, you will very quickly be able to determine whether it's a one-size-fits-all product for bronzing and contouring.

Here are some simple, Lazy Perfection contouring steps:
- Draw a line underneath the cheekbone (from the center of the ear cartilage to the hollow of the cheek, staying in line with the corner of the mouth), and then blend away any edges. This will create the appearance of hollowed cheeks and lifted cheekbones.
- Draw narrow, vertical lines down the front and sides of the neck,

on either side of the Adam's apple, and blend well so that you look elongated and not striped.

- Drag a brush with contour powder along the bottom edge of the jawline and slightly underneath. This defines the shape, makes it look distinct and separate from the neck, conceals any loose skin under the chin and makes it appear more firm and lifted.
- Contour into the socket line of the eye to create the impression that the lid is longer and taller.
- Buff color into the temples and around the hairline to slim and shorten the forehead.

See, the dark side isn't so bad. Now we can punctuate our makeup with the opposite effect.

Dots and Dashes

Lazy Perfection fans want to be noticed and admired, of course, but not because they have spectacular, flawless makeup. They simply understand the power that comes with confidence, self-awareness, and ease. And that's why one of the very first Lazy Perfection Punctuation Marks is called Strategic Highlighting, a way to add dashes and dots of light to the most flattering points on the face.

Highlighting is simply the way in which light gets attracted to and then reflected away from your skin to lend radiance to the complexion. Matte highlighters—those without any shimmer in them—bounce light away by virtue of being light in color, resulting in a slower reflection. Shimmery highlighters bounce light away from the skin fast because of the flashes of metallic in their small particles. It's actually a pretty simple concept.

The strategic part comes in when you figure out how to harness that light and how it can best flatter your features.

- Cheeks look more lifted.
- Skin looks more hydrated.
- Eyes look more open and bright.
- Lips look fuller.
- The nose looks slimmer.

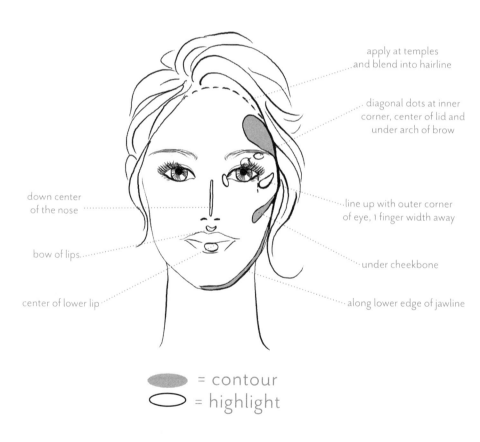

apply at temples and blend into hairline

diagonal dots at inner corner, center of lid and under arch of brow

down center of the nose

line up with outer corner of eye, 1 finger width away

bow of lips

under cheekbone

center of lower lip

along lower edge of jawline

⬬ = contour
⬭ = highlight

Cheeks, Comma, Glowing Cheeks

It always makes me laugh a little when I read in the magazines or blogs that "radiant skin" is a big beauty trend for fall, spring, or whenever. Because, like, when isn't fresh, youthful skin in style? Dull skin as a trend has never, to my knowledge, been a smashing success. It's classic to have glowing, bright skin, and a little touch of highlighter can be a gorgeous enhancement.

The trendy part of highlighter has been more about the degree of reflection on the cheeks, and that nuclear waste look has been "in" for quite some time now. Just to be clear, we're not going for that YouTube Beauty Guru level of highlighting here, ladies. My approach is much more subtle and understated.

Cream formulas tend to be the ones that blend the most easily and meld with the skin, which is what gives the appearance of hydration in addition to a luminous reflection of light. Powders are fine for unlined skin, but for the rest of us, they may sit on top of the skin and accentuate flaws. Obviously, my preference is for creams or liquids. It looks most natural to select a highlighter color that is in the same general tone as your skin—peachy/gold for warm complexions, pink/pearly tones for cool tones, ivory/beige for neutral tones.

- Highlighter should be placed in a short stripe at the very top of the cheeks (see diagram on page 148), lined up vertically with the outer corner of the eye about one horizontal finger's width underneath. If it's placed closer than one finger's width away, it will call attention to even the most miniuscule of fine lines and can even make the eyes look puffy or swollen.

- Highlighter may also be wrapped from the top of the cheek up around the top of the brow, in a small, inverted C-shape. This gives the impression that that whole area of the face is lifted and taut, and that the skin is hydrated and dewy.

- If you have deeper lines around the eyes or on the cheeks, you should select a matte highlighter. Shimmery particles can sink to the bottom of those lines and act like a beacon, calling even more attention to them.
- Highlighter should not be blended into the apple of the cheeks or anywhere close to the nose, as it may float on top of the pores and magnify them.

Exclamation Point Eyes

When highlighting the eyes, think of creating an upward diagonal line of light from the inner corner to under the arch of the brow. Using this technique, you are strategically drawing a line of light to create the illusion of lift. These steps can be done on their own or all together, as you prefer, and if you stick with a sheer, neutral beige color, it won't distract from the rest of your makeup or look too obvious.

- Apply a small amount of highlighter just around your tear duct, on the inner corner of the eye. This makes them look soft and dewy.
- Apply a dab of highlighter on the very center of your eyelid, immediately above the iris. Every time you blink, you will get a subtle flash of light that makes the eyes look bright and awake.
- Add a dab of highlighter just underneath the arch of the brow. This make the brow look higher, which gives the overall impression that the eyes are big and lifted.
- With a thin, flat makeup brush, draw a small line of highlighter up from the outer corners of the eyes, aimed at the temples. This will make the corners of the eyes look bright and lifted.

Pout Parentheses

Highlighting is actually a really easy way to give the lips a little more oomph, without looking like you just got back from a plastic surgery vacation to South America. But when I say parentheses, I do not mean the side to side parentheses (like in the nasal labial folds—ugh—still the worst anatomical name ever). I mean using highlighting as a way to frame out the top and the bottom of your lips.

- A small dab of highlighter in the bow of the lips can make them look poutier, but a word to the wise: taking that dab too far up can make you look like you've got a drippy nose situation, which, as far as I know, has never been greeted with cries of "Hot damn, that's so sexy!"

- A tiny pat of highlighter in the center of the lower lip creates the look of fullness. This can be done over or under your other lip products.

- A small, thin line of highlighter drawn diagonally up from the corners of the mouth creates the appearance of lift, although this is better done with matte highlighter, as shimmer on that part of the face would be too obvious and detectable.

Vertical Dash

Finally, if you want to make your nose look slimmer and higher, drawing a thin line of highlighter down the center, from bridge to tip, creates a thin ridge of light that makes the nose look more streamlined. While not found in actual punctuation, a vertical dash is simply a visual separator—a way to break up the space. I would caution you not to use products that are too shimmery, as they can make your skin look slick instead of satiny—totally the opposite effect you would want. That's also why I don't recommend using highlighter on the forehead or chin—it doesn't make sense to me that you would want to use shimmer on areas of the face that produce oils naturally and already have a reflective sheen.

Lash But Not Least . . .

Now, I know this is going to be a controversial recommendation, which is why I have included it in the Lazy Perfection Punctuation chapter and not as a part of the Lazy Perfection Simple, Sophisticated, or Sexy Tracks.

- I believe in the power of eyelash curlers.
- I believe that they can completely transform the eyes.
- But I don't believe that everyone can or should use one.

TPW was probably born with naturally dark, thick curly lashes—her eyes always look so open and awake. Think of it this way—when your lashes are straight, they act like a canopy for the eyes, creating shade underneath. But when they have been curled, they are up and out of the way so that the light can get to your eyes. It's an instant eye lift, and one that I find particularly helpful when I wake up puffy and inflamed.

So, consider eyelash curlers unless you:

1) Have TPW quality lashes that are naturally curly

or

2) Have an aversion to putting small implements near your eyes (which many women do).

Eyelash curlers are a strong ! for your eye makeup application. Fine. Yes. They look like mini torture devices. If you have been pinched by one before, the chances are good that you won't want to try it again. If you have heard horror stories of people losing their lashes from using one, I understand your skepticism. But I want you to keep an open mind.

The Shape of Things

If you have pinched yourself with a lash curler, it's most likely because you were using one that's the wrong shape for your eyes. Who knew that lash curlers come in different sizes and shapes, right? But they do. You need to find one that hugs your lash line, where the edge of it lies flush against the roots of your lashes. If it doesn't, it will grab the skin on your lid and ouch! That does indeed hurt like crazy.

Step 1—Find a curler that fits. Shiseido is great for women with deep-set or hooded eyes, Surratt Beauty works for almond eyes, and Kevyn Aucoin is suitable for just about everyone else.

Feel Your Way

Step 2—Learn how to use it by feel and not by sight. When it's placed in just the right spot, with the upper edge of the curler resting on top of the roots of your lashes and the lower, rubbery edge supporting the roots underneath, you should feel a slight tug when you squeeze. If you don't feel that tug at your roots, you are too far up on your lashes and will get a bend mark. Gently wiggle the curler down to where it's hugging the roots, and try to squeeze again.

Hot and Pulsing

Do I have your attention with this caption? Good—because listen up. There are the right ways to use your lash curler, and there are plenty of wrong ways.

I don't believe in the technique in which you squeeze at the roots, then move up to the middle of the lashes and then closer to the tips—that's a lot of extra work and leaves you vulnerable to crimp marks. Just a few pulses at the roots of the lashes will curl them up, without bending them. I usually count to about five pulses, but for clients who are just getting comfortable with a curler, I find that counting backward from five makes it a little more tolerable.

A curler can be slightly warmed up before use to help hold the curl. Contrary to popular belief, it does not need to be blasted with a hair dryer to build the heat—you can simply rub it back and forth on a washcloth a few times. Lash curlers are metal, so you just need to take the chill off—blasting them with hot air and then putting it on your lid can actually burn your skin. Not worth the risk. Battery heated lash curlers are a waste of time and money because they don't really work. It's a bummer because it sounds like such a good idea.

Curl Then Coat

Mascara should absolutely not be applied before you curl your lashes. The waxy coating can stick to your lashes and pull them out. If this has happened to you, I understand that you are traumatized. If you tempt fate and apply mascara first, make sure you WIPE OFF EXCESS from your curler after every single use. Even eyeliner that builds up on your curler can stick to your lashes and pull them out.

If your lashes are stubbornly straight and don't hold that curl well, go over each eye twice, and then apply a volumizing mascara right away, wiggling the applicator back and forth right at the root of the lashes. Thickening (aka volumizing) mascaras tend to have heavier waxes in them, so they'll support the curl better than thinner, lengthening mascaras can. I have yet to come across a curling mascara that works well, I'm afraid. I keep holding out hope, though.

Oh, Snap

A client called me not too long ago, totally flipped out that her lash curler had snapped off her lashes. Like a big chunk of them. I would be freaking out, too.

The rubber pads on eyelash curlers start to break down over time and with repeated rigorous use. If you see an indentation or well start to form in it, replace it right away. That indentation or well acts just like a mini lash guillotine, and it's just not a humane way to treat your lashes.

Hyphen Hands

And finally, your hands and nails are important to your overall beauty look because not only can they blab your true age to anyone who looks at you below the neck, but so many of us use them to gesticulate and express ourselves, so they do attract attention.

Honestly, the best thing you can do for your hands is apply moisturizer every time you wash them. It will seal in any tiny droplets of water that have been left behind, keeping the thin skin from looking crepey. This is something that doesn't require a big investment—any old hand cream will do.

I also suggest making the backs of your hands the last stop on your skincare routine. Leftover serum on your fingers? Rub it onto the backs of your hands. The same goes for any other products like antioxidants and Retinol. It might take a little extra time to see results because they're a skincare afterthought and not getting the full treatment (which, of course, you can give them, if you like), but what you'll end up with is fewer age spots, plumper skin, and less visible veins. Oh, how I hate those veins.

Cuticle Colons

It's true. Raggedy, ripped, dried-out cuticles just don't scream "fresh!"
or "chic!" If you can apply cuticle oil over the course of the day,
congratulations—that's impressive effort that I can't seem to muster.
What I do find to be Lazy Perfection nail bed care is simply applying a
little coconut oil, Aquaphor or Vaseline on top of them at bedtime. It
holds in moisture and softens the skin while you're asleep. There's nothing
more Lazy Perfection than skincare, or in this case cuticle care, in your
sleep.

Nails, Nails, Nails

I am going to confess that one of my least favorite things to do is a get a
manicure or do my nails. I know that so many women love it and find it
relaxing, but to me, it's an hour (or more) out of my day that I can rarely
afford to take.

But, I do think that having polished, well-kept nails is one of the more
important Lazy Perfection punctuation marks, mostly because chipped
polish and ragged edges look the opposite of fresh, modern, youthful,
and put together. TPW would never be out and about with haggard-
looking cuticles and choppy, bitten tips, right?

Fortunately, there are some very cool spray-on nail polishes now
that are gloriously imprecise in application, but perfectly smooth in
finish. The sprays from Nails, Inc. are particularly easy to use—and
you know how I feel about precision and Lazy Perfection. They are
ARCHENEMIES. These spray on like a hot mess, but then any color
that doesn't land directly on your nails simply washes away. It's Lazy
Perfection genius.

I am also a big fan of gel polish, which leaves you with a no-chip finish for up to two to three weeks. Now, there's some controversy about using UV light to set the gel into a hard finish, as there may be potential skin health risks, but plenty of gels now only require natural sunlight. Polish that holds its shine, doesn't chip, dent, or smudge is the DEFINITION of Lazy Perfection. Hallelujah.

So, whether you want to put an !, ?, or . . . into your beauty routine, you have lots of options to add a little somethin' somethin'. Just remember what you are trying to convey. A suggestive glance, a seductive pout, a whimsical come hither . . . or even just a hint of a "Damn, I look great today!" is enough to amp up your Lazy Perfection Look.

CHAPTER ELEVEN

A Hairstory Lesson

REMEMBER WAY BACK IN THE INTRODUCTION WHEN I TOLD YOU that Lazy Perfection is about getting all the aspects of your personal appearance together in one cohesive, flattering, simplified way? Well, now it's time for the rubber to meet the road, because we're stepping away from makeup and moving on to hair. But before we do, we need to take a lesson from history and explore our hairstory, because when it comes to our hair, where we came from is as important as where we're going.

Ancient Hairstory

Our hair changes over time, both in color and texture. Many of us have heat styled, chemically treated, changed colors, tried new styles and lengths, experienced thinning, or have simply gotten into a rut where it doesn't look as fresh and youthful as it used to. Remember those pictures of you as a child, and your hair was all soft and shiny and the color was totally angelic? Wouldn't it be great to go back to that? Too bad life, hormones, pollution, the whims of fashion—and, you know, the lack of a time machine—all get in the way of us really ever getting back there. Sigh. That naturally soft, healthy hair is ancient history.

Our hair can have even more of an impact on how we feel than our makeup—we've all experienced our fair share of "Bad Hair Days," and know what a total, debilitating drag they can be. The care and keeping of our hair is definitely critical to how it looks and, in turn, how we feel, but let's take a look at how it works with our makeup and fashion choices. Of course I want to share with you my Lazy Perfection approach to nourishing, protecting, and styling your hair, but I also want to fill you in on some Lazy Perfection hair-styling secrets that are going to change the way you look at yourself.

The Renaissance Period

Everyone knows that the color of your hair can perk up your complexion and be a great rejuvenator, a beauty renaissance, but what we don't often consider is how our makeup needs to be calibrated to go along with it. Eyes are always eyes, and the shadow and liner colors that make them pop are a constant, but when it comes to the complexion and lips, it may be worth bumping up your bronzer or modifying your colors a bit. There are millions of different tones of blonde, brunette, and redhead, but here's a quick breakdown of the makeup that will be the most flattering on them.

As a quick refresher, just remember that "warm" means any color that has hints of orange, red, or yellow in it. Think of a fire and the colors you see in the flames. "Cool" means colors that could put out the fire, like water or sand, anything with white, silver, brown, blue, or gray undertones.

There are more shades of hair color than there are flavors of jelly beans, but here are the ones that are most commonly seen.

The Cool Blondes

- **Platinum** (Think Marilyn Monroe or Gwen Stefani)—Cool and pale, with a white or creamy white base. Makeup for platinums is most flattering in complementary cool, soft, pearly tones and with a little warmth added in from a subtle, pale bronzer. Lips should have a dash of color to them, like a soft pink, so that you don't look washed out. Dark liner is a great contrast on platinum blondes, but can look heavy, so stick with gray, brown, and navy instead of black.

Neutral Blondes

- **Beige** (Think Reese Witherspoon, Kate Hudson, or Amanda Seyfried)—Beige blonde is like creamy coffee or a yummy faded cashmere cardigan. Beige blondes can generally wear both warm, peachy tones and an array of soft, neutral pink tones. Playing up the cheeks gives life to the complexion of a beige blonde.

The Warm Blondes

- **Honey/Golden** (Think Jennifer Aniston or Gwyneth Paltrow)—Warm yellow–toned blonde is the color of, you guessed it, honey. Avoid blue-based makeup colors and opt instead for soft browns, peaches, and corals. Purple-y colors are not flattering on honey blondes, and neither are fuchsias or anything too blue. Extra bronzer looks great on honey and golden blondes.
- **Caramel** (Think Ciara or JLo) Warm, medium blonde, the color of melted caramel. Monochromatic makeup looks great on caramel blondes, keeping the cheeks and lips in the same bare caramel or golden family, with a little extra liner around the eyes for a touch of glamour.

The Cool Brunettes

- **Ash** (Think Sarah Jessica Parker or Mila Kunis) Ashy hair has very little warmth/red/gold in it and can be light, medium, or dark in tone. It's often referred to as mousy brown but with a little additional makeup can be absolutely gorgeous. Ashy-haired gals will always benefit from warming up their complexion with bronzer and adding warm rose colors to their cheeks and lips.

- **Mahogany** (Think Kris or Kendall Jenner)—Mahogany brown hair has lots of blue, almost black undertones to it. Mahogany gals look lovely with pale, radiant skin, sheer but bright pink blush, plenty of eyeliner, and a lip color that's a couple of shades lighter or deeper than their natural color. Makeup that's too bland will dull and fade the features.

Neutral Brunettes

- **Bronde**—(Think Gisele Bündchen or Drew Barrymore)—This is a natural brunette base color with enough blonde highlights to appear blonde. It's a totally neutral color that looks good with bronzer, peaches, and pinks. The blonde accents reflect the light beautifully and make the skin look luminous, so not much makeup is required to boost the radiance of the complexion.

The Warm Brunettes

- **Golden or Caramel** (think Jessica Alba or Jessica Biel)—Cousins to brondes, golden brunettes have a brown base color with warm, golden highlights. Bronzer picks up those highlights and makes the complexion look luminous, and warm peach-, apricot-, or coral-based colors will set off the complexion even more.
- **Chocolate** (Think Katie Holmes or Sandra Bullock)—Chocolate brunettes have a darker brown base color with subtle pieces of warm, chestnut brown woven through. Chocolate is a balance of warm and cool tones, so makeup can be warm or cool in tone as well. Whichever

direction you go, calling attention to the eyes by adding additional eyeliner and mascara will be very flattering.

The Cool Reds . . . Just Kidding . . .there are no cool reds. They are all warm.

For all redheads, colors should be kept warm—in the peach, apricot, and brick families, but lip colors with cooler berry or pink tones can also be lovely. Light redheads should use light makeup colors with a little extra blush on the cheeks to give life to the complexion, and darker redheads should add a stronger pop of color on their cheeks and lips as well. Bronzer all the way around, though—it sets off freckles and pale skin in a particularly gorgeous way, and anything with a luminous or reflective finish is also lovely on freckly skin.

- Strawberry Blonde (aka Ginger)—Think Nicole Kidman or Jessica Chastain—Blonde with tinges of red or orange in it.
- Copper—Think Amy Adams—Like a shiny, new penny, copper is a bright but light red.
- Auburn—Think Susan Sarandon or Julianne Moore—Auburn is a mix of red and brown and can be light, medium, or dark in tone.
- Fiery (aka Cinnamon, aka Bright Copper)—Think Christina Hendricks or Lucille Ball—Bright red hair is medium in tone and has a slight golden undertone.
- Chestnut—Think Julia Roberts—A base of brown hair with a strong accent of rich, dark red. Chestnut brunettes look best in rich, warm colors like apricot or rose.
- Dark Cherry (Think Sharon Osbourne)—Cherry red is a mix of dark blue/brunette and dark red, and cool-toned makeup is the most flattering with it, like berry tones.

The Grays—obviously, these colors are all cool. Despite the fact that a little bronzer will make the skin look fresher and more youthful, the rest of the makeup palette can be slightly warm or slightly cool, depending on personal preference. A soft-apricot or warm-rose cheek and lip will always be lovely, but berry and pink tones work well, too. What doesn't work on gray, silver, or salt-and-pepper ladies? Anything too orange, brick, or copper in tone.

Think Jamie Lee Curtis, Helen Mirren, and, fictional or not, Miranda Priestly (*The Devil Wears Prada*).

On the Wrong Side of Hairstory

Grown out roots used to put us on the wrong side of hairstory, acting as very clear proof that we're not naturally the color we appear. I have personally been almost every color under the sun, from platinum to red to dark brown, and now I'm edging ever closer to gray. The one thing I can tell you is that the relationship between your hair color and your brow color is super important. You can actually make your hair color look more flattering and chic simply by adjusting the color of your eyebrows.

- **Blondes:** Try to more or less match the color of your roots when filling in your brows. So naturally, as the roots get longer and darker between coloring, the brows should get a little darker as well. This will limit the attention your roots get because they won't stand out quite as much.

- **Light to medium brunettes:** The brows should be kept at around the same color as your lightest pieces of hair. If the lighter pieces are warm, then use warm tones in the brows, and vice versa for cool tones.

- **Redheads:** The brows of most natural redheads are generally lighter or darker than their hair. Look for products that have a light brown base with some slight red mixed in. A too-red color will look clownish and unnatural, and a dark, ashy color will be out of balance.

- **Gray:** Stay in the cool-toned family, looking to original hair color for inspiration. For former blondes, look for light, taupey colors; former brunettes should stay in the soft brown range, and former redheads should look for a golden blonde color. It's a statement to wear a very dark brow with gray hair, but if that's your original hair color, then by all means keep your brows dark, but just use a light touch when filling them in. You don't want to go down that Groucho Marx road, if you know what I mean.

Honestly, there might not be any better way to turn back the clock than to add just a few face-framing highlights or lowlights to your hair. They attract and reflect light differently than an all-over color will, and can add radiance that wasn't previously there.

The cut you get is important, too, because the shape and length of your hair need to work with your features. There's no point in going to your stylist asking for Blake Lively's haircut if it's something that really won't flatter you— you just need to be armed with a little information so that when you do get your hair done, you have an idea of what will work best for you.

Bygone Bangs

You've heard the expression Bangs or Botox, right? Well, I can't say that I think bangs are for everyone, but they certainly do offer the advantage of covering any forehead lines that might be bothering you, which is a Lazy Perfection approach for sure. Bangs work best on women who have a long forehead or a high hairline, meaning that if you break the face into equal thirds from the hairline to the chin, the forehead has extra space. Try this.

- Flatten out your hand with your fingers together and then turn it horizontally so it's flat to your face, with the bottom of your pinky even with the bottom of your chin.

- Stack your other hand horizontally on top of it and then stack your bottom hand on top of that.
- If there's more than a finger's width of space between your top hand and your hairline, you're a candidate for bangs.

Side swept, heavy, feathery—that all depends on your hair texture and what's in fashion, but assuming you can make it work, it would look good on you.

Part of the Past

Sometimes, your hair will decide for you where it wants to be parted, depending on whether you have a cowlick or a natural wave. And if that's the case, you just have to go with it, because there's no use fighting nature—that's not the Lazy Perfection way. But if you've always wondered whether you should switch up your part, let me give you these little tips to help you decide. Just remember that part placement is impacted by trends, so you do have to be sure that you are embracing a look that is current, not a part of the past.

You need to consider the angles on your face and the symmetry of your features. Models always look good in photos because their faces are perfectly symmetrical, but the rest of us mere mortals typically have some features that are off-center or out of balance. Here are the Lazy Perfection ways to get them balanced again.

- A center part will work well if you have a round or square jawline because it draws the eye down and creates the impression that there's more length down the sides of your face.
- A side part looks good on long, oval, or narrow faces because it creates

the illusion of more width across the cheekbones. This is also good for anyone who wants to hide crepey or aging skin on the cheeks and along the jawline, since it softly frames the face instead of creating the strong, straight lines a center part does. Those strong, straight lines call too much attention to the contrast against the softening of our skin.

- **An off-center part,** just slightly to one side or another, is flattering on anyone with a tall or broad forehead, a strong jawline, or asymmetrical eyes because it cuts into the harsh angles, making them appear softer, less pronounced, and more evenly weighted.

Length Lore

I never want to hear anyone say ever again that there's a point at which women age out of long hair. Seriously? As long as it's healthy, flattering, and in fashion, then there's absolutely no reason that a "mature" woman should have to cut off all her hair. It's the hair equivalent to nude lipstick—there's a style that will look good on everyone, as long as you're working with a smooth, healthy base. Hair length goes in and out of style, so as we age, we need to make adjustments to avoid looking dated and old-fashioned. If you've had the exact same hairstyle for thirty years, then maybe it's time to reevaluate. That doesn't mean that you have to go from Christie Brinkley to your high school librarian (no disrespect to high school librarians—just stereotyping for illustrative purposes), but it does mean that shaking things up once in a while can be exciting, and revitalizing.

Long hair has the advantage of drawing the eye down. It can make you look taller and leaner, as long as it's shaped and parted in a way that flatters your features. I particularly love long hair with a V-neck top, which is one of the Lazy Perfection fashion picks we'll talk about in the next chapter.

Midlength hair also comes in and out of fashion, but hair that falls somewhere between the collarbones and the chin moves beautifully and frames out the décolletage and neck, adding the look of length and a certain gracefulness to the wearer. Call it a Lob, call it a Bob—whatever you want. It's the bronzer of hair lengths—versatile and flattering on pretty much everyone.

Short hair is the red lipstick of hair styles. There might be a style that will be flattering for everyone, but not everyone should try it. It takes confidence to rock a pixie, and unless it works with your hair texture and your personal style, it can throw off your whole beauty game. Remember that confidence is the key to Lazy Perfection—if you feel good about how you look, then you'll look good. Going from long or midlength to short hair is a big step that can throw even the most confident women into a state of hair-style catatonia.

The Up-Do Era

Updos. Oh, updos. They are the antithesis of Lazy Perfection. So much time and effort and spray and pinning goes into getting them in place, and then once they are in place, they can look less natural than a spray tan on a politician. They can look as dated as an era long since passed.

Let me put in plainly: I'm not a fan of the updo. For special occasions, I prefer a softer, looser, deconstructed look. Hair that's touchable, not helmet-esque.

In truth, my preferred Lazy Perfection updo, if it can even be counted as one, is the humble ponytail. Placed just right, it can make the cheekbones look higher, the neck look longer, and the jawline look firmer. And pretty much anyone can do it in the comfort of her own home, depending on how long their hair is and how short their layers are.

To get the most flattering look, simply brush your hair up and back so that it's in the same line and angle as your cheekbones. Any higher and you'll look like your face has been pulled taut, and any lower and it can actually make your features appear droopy. But placed just right, a ponytail is a hairdo face-lift.

Of Dubious Descent

I need to give you some bad news. Unlike your skin, your hair is not a living part of your system. We treat it like it's alive, but in truth, the living part of our hair follicles is found underneath our scalp. By the time it breaks through, it's already dead. So, our hair is pretty much a zombie—undead.

But the good news here is that, as with skin, we can fake the look of life and luster. And we can do it in a relatively easy way. The haircare industry is every bit as much of a behemoth as skincare and cosmetics, maybe even more so because men take care of their hair as well, and it can be every bit as overwhelming. So in this chapter, I'm going to help you figure out what exactly it is you'll need to get on the best Lazy Perfection Haircare Track for you.

The Reformation

But first, let's talk food. We all know how important it is to eat lots of veggies and to limit our intake of simple carbohydrates (so sad), but I want to talk about it in terms of how it affects your hair. Yes, your hair. If you reform your diet, you can reform your hair.

Believe me, I know it's hard to eat perfectly all the time and follow all the rules, especially because it seems like those rules change every day. Eat avocado. Don't eat corn. East as much bacon as you want. Wait, don't eat bacon, but do eat cheese. Wait, cheese is bad but yogurt is okay. It's constantly confusing.

I fall on and off the nutrition wagon all the time, cycling in and out of being wheat-free (it makes my eyelids puffy), sugar-free (it makes me break out), dairy-free (don't ask . . . too embarrassing), and carb-free (makes me bloated). I'm "good" for a few weeks, maybe a few months, and then bam—one bite of an onion ring or a spoonful of coffee ice cream, and I fall off the wagon hard and back into the arms of my irresistible lover, chips. There is no food more glorious in its perfection than the chip—potato, tortilla . . . it doesn't matter, I don't discriminate. I am poly-chip-amorous.

Despite the intoxicating endorphin rush that comes from cheating on kale with Cheetos, I'm not telling you anything new when I say that junk food is not good for us—our body, skin, or hair. Obviously, the food we eat impacts the way our bodies function and how our skin behaves. Our skin is a living organ, the wrapping paper around our internal organ system, intertwined and copacetic. It's (theoretically) easy to take care of our skin by eating well, avoiding inflammatory foods, and drinking plenty of water. And, while we slather on expensive creams, luxuriate in facials, and hunt for nontoxic products, we often don't make the conscious connection between what we eat and our hair.

By the time our hair breaks through our scalp, it's already dead, but we treat it like it's alive, and have the expectation that it will respond as though it's alive. The only way to really and truly ensure that our hair is healthy from its core is to nourish it before it springs forth, and then to manage the aftermath.

So before we get down to the meat and potatoes of how you can Lazy Perfectionize your hair routine, we need to prepare for the . . .

Age of Enlightenment

The only living part of our hair is under our scalp—the visible part, the part we badly mistreat with heat styling, chemicals, and environmental stressors, is where we need to get enlightened.

Haircare companies toy with us. They use all kinds of fancy marketing speak to let us think that we can grow more hair, or thicker hair. That's simply not the case. As with our brows and lashes, we are born with exactly the number of follicles we will always have, so we are never going to be able to have more, and even though we can chemically alter the texture of our hair to make it straighter or curlier, we cannot actually grow more follicles. Haircare marketing people everywhere are grimacing at the debunking of this myth, but that's the real truth.

What we can do to help our hair is strengthen each follicle and support the natural growth and shedding cycles so that we aren't losing all our hair at once, without having new hair at the ready to come right in and replace it.

Hunters and Gatherers

There is very little that we can do that's better for our hair (and our skin) than to eat well. Not groundbreaking news here. But, if grocery shopping, cooking, and cleaning up aren't for you, then there's an even simpler, even lazier route you can take. You don't need to be like ancient man and head out to hunt and gather. You can take the Lazy Perfection approach.

Be a Pill Popper

Obviously, it's better to get your nutrients from food, but short of getting over to your local farmers' market, you can supplement your nutritional intake with vitamins. From a Lazy Perfection standpoint, I am all over the concept of taking supplements and have personally found them to be downright impactful. But, to be clear, taking them is the Lazy part . . . getting to the point where you can see the results takes consistency, time, and patience. A vitamin regimen is a time investment—there are no overnight fixes. Hair grows an average of one-quarter inch per month, so it could easily be six to eight months before you see any appreciable change. Beautiful hair is worth the wait, so making a commitment to a vitamin routine is of the essence.

Obviously, eating well is important here, too, but targeted vitamin formulas for skincare and haircare are both plentiful and readily available. They are also targeted so that you can determine quite easily the best vitamins for you and your specific concerns.

Biotin: Biotin is a Vitamin-B complex that helps with elasticity and the production of keratin, which is the very core of healthy hair. It is a BFF to hair that is fragile and prone to breakage. Biotin can also be found in foods such as lentils, brown rice, green peas, and oats—just in case you feel like cooking.

Vitamin A: A potent antioxidant (the same one found in Retin-A), Vitamin A helps to produce sebum on the scalp and hair, which improves elasticity and shine, but you must follow the dosage and directions carefully, as too much Vitamin A can cause dizziness, headaches, or nausea. You can also eat your Vitamin A in the form of peaches, spinach, and carrots.

Vitamin E: Vitamin E is another antioxidant and can help prevent free-radical damage that comes from environmental damage related to pollution or sun exposure. It speeds up the body's circulation and intake of oxygen, which may also help prevent hair loss. Vitamin E can be found in beans, soybeans, leafy greens, and nuts.

Omega-3 Fatty Acids: It's all in the name. The "good" fat in these omega acids is what gives hair and skin a natural glow, and their anti-inflammatory properties help with skin conditions like acne and psoriasis. Omega-3s—from salmon, anchovies, sardines, and other oily fish, olive oil, and avocadoes—also strengthen and help to protect the hair against breakage.

There are all sorts of new vitamin drinks you can add to your beauty routine, if drinking your nutrition seems simpler to you. It's all about finding a plan, and then sticking with it.

The Inquisition

Now you have a sense of what dietary supplements and foods can help with hair care—but what do we do about all the hair that didn't have the advantages of good nutrition and vitamin supplements? And how can we take care of it without spending precious time and money to make it look un-undead or living in the past? Well, let's start off by assessing the situation, going through an inquisition, if you will.

WHAT'S YOUR HAIR TYPE?

- Normal—You can wash and go, don't need a lot of products to get control, and don't overly suffer from frizz, flyaways, oily roots, split ends, or breakage. Not sure why this hair type would be called "normal," to be honest, since it seems more like the exception.

- Dry—Your hair often lacks luster and shine, is prone to breakage or damage and drinks up conditioner like a sponge sops up water.
- Oily—You can't go more than a day without washing, your roots become slick and sticky easily and too much product makes your hair lie down flatter than a slug on a sidewalk.
- Fine—Each individual strand of your hair is super thin, although you may have lots and lots of strands.
- Coarse—You are prone to frizz and kink and spend a good amount of time trying to coax your hair into submission.
- Damaged—You color or chemically treat your hair, it snaps when you brush it, your ends are split, and you frequently battle frizz and flyaways.

What's your haircare INTENTION?

Like, what do you really hope to achieve when you are getting ready every day?
- Do you want your hair to grow faster?
- Shine brighter?
- Look thicker and fuller?
- Bounce and swing?
- Or just cooperate better?
- Do you want to get out the door faster?
- Do you want to look more polished and put together?
- Do you want to refresh and update your look?
- Do you want to heal the damage?

As with skincare, I am going to show you three different tracks you can get on to address your haircare needs—a SIMPLE one, a SOPHISTICATED one, and a SEXY one. You'll just need to assess, which is going to get you closest to your objective and work best for your hair type, lifestyle, personal style, and technical skill set.

Yes—the technical skill set is SUPER important when it comes to hair. It's not like applying makeup or creams, where your entire workspace is in front of you. With hair, there's a whole lot of backstage action going on, and we would certainly all benefit from octopus arms and a three-, four-, or five-way mirror. In fact, the first thing I would recommend you get is a three-way mirror, or at the very least, a large handheld mirror that will give you a large enough reflection to see what's really happening on the dark side of the moon. The teeny-tiny mirror in your blush compact is really not going to cut it.

A Brush with Fate

You should also make sure that you get the right tools to do your hair. Like makeup brushes, it's best to be intentional about the shape and texture of your tools so that they will give you desirable results. And like makeup brushes, there are hundreds of different options out there. Here's really what you need to know:

- Round "radial" brushes—The larger the barrel, the more volume you will get. The smaller the barrel, the more curl you will get. It's virtually impossible to dry your hair stick straight with a round brush, but you can get a smooth, voluminous result. If your hair is on the fine side, look for a round brush that has a mixture of short and long bristles to make sure that every hair gets gripped.

- Half-radial brushes—Ideal for getting either volume or tension at the root for lift and smoothing. Half radials are the workhorse of hairbrushes and are suitable for just about anyone.

- Flat or paddle brushes—The flatter the brush, the flatter the hair. Large paddles work best on long hair since they have more surface area to drag the hair through. It's extremely difficult to get a curl or wave with a flat paddle brush.

- Vented brush—The little holes in the underside of the brush allow for better airflow with heat styling and a faster drying process but generally are not suitable for adding shape to the hair, since they have very few bristles to offer any control.

- Thermal brushes—Thermal brushes have a core made from metal or ceramic that holds on to the heat from your dryer and distributes it back into the hair evenly and without damage. Think of them like a brick pizza oven—it's the secondary heat that helps it get cooked faster and more evenly.

- Natural bristles—Like the natural bristles on a makeup brush, they will absorb a certain amount of the oil from your hair and your products, redistributing them in with every stroke and leaving your hair shiny and glossy.

- Nylon bristles—The biggest thing to consider with nylon or plastic bristles is that they can melt under extreme heat, so caution is required during heat styling. Plenty of brushes have a mix of nylon and natural bristles, so just be aware when you make your selection so that you are using it with the appropriate amount of heat.

JUST STOP thinking that any old brush will do when you're combing through wet hair. The basic rule of thumb to avoid snapping delicate, wet strands is to choose a brush with bristles that don't feel prickly on the palm of your hand. If they're prickly, they're not smooth, and if they're not smooth, they'll snag.

Making History.

You know my feelings on the Lazy Perfection Tracks by now—you can mix and match them, change them up, depending on what you're wearing, where you're going, or what you're doing—but my objective with hair care, as with skincare and makeup, is to show you how you can streamline your routine and still get consistently lovely results. By making a few small shifts in your hair care routine, your "hairstory" will be one for the ages.

Obviously, washing is going to be the first step everyone should take. But, unlike your face which needs to be washed every day at bedtime without fail, hair should be washed only as necessary. You don't want to strip away all the oils on your scalp that help your hair look alive. Removing all those oils will cause your hair to rebel—getting dry, brittle, and frizzy over time. Of course, too much oil isn't a good thing, either, so you'll have to determine how long you can go between washes.

And conditioning. It goes without saying that conditioner is essential for adding moisture back into your hair, smoothing down the hair cuticle that's been roughed up by washing, and protecting it from future damage. But it's important to choose a conditioner that's consistent with your hair intention and then make sure that it's applied correctly. As with makeup, start slowly and add more if you feel you need it, and avoid applying conditioner to your roots as it can weight hair down and leave you looking limp and greasy. It's like applying hydrating foundation on oily skin—you're just going to end up with a slick, slippery mess.

And now you need to know all the other hair care options available to you. They are the hair equivalents of Retinols, antioxidants, and AHAs. There is an enormous menu of choices out there, so let's take a look at some of them and then determine which one is right for you.

The Gilded Age

Everyone can use a little extra hydration and nourishment, since those are the primary ways you can make your hair look more shiny and radiant, as though it has been gilded.

- Deep conditioner—Once a week, once a month, whenever you can get around to it, using a creamy or oily product to smooth rough follicles and improve texture will make a difference, albeit not a long-term one. No matter what you read or hear, there are no long-term or cumulative benefits to deep conditioning, which is why you need to do it repeatedly.
- Serums and oils—You have to think of these exactly the same way you would think of serums and oils for your skin in that they should be used to treat specific issues. Overnight serum and oil treatments for hair are attractive ways to nourish, and they can also be helpful in protecting hair during chemical treatment services at the salon.

The Control Chronicles

Here are the products you can use to maintain control, and chronicle for posterity your soon-to-be many good hair days.

- Gel—Gels create a film that dries in between each strand of hair and essentially glues them together. They may contain alcohol and even plastics, which is what can leave that hard, crunchy feel. They're best suited to hair that needs texture with control, like for curls or a slicked-back look.
- Hair cream—Hair cream is gel's cooler, younger cousin. It gives the same weight and definition to hair that gel does, but without leaving that crunchy feeling when it dries. Ideal for natural, textured, or curly hair.
- Hair spray—The key to successful hair spray selection is to know how much hold you need. Light hold helps with flyaways but keeps softness and movement in the rest of the hair; medium hold has a little more density; and firm hold is industrial strength, for updos.
- Finishing spray—If you've ever wondered about the difference

between finishing spray and hair spray, let me put it in skincare terms—everyone can benefit from a basic moisturizer, but serums target your specific issues. Same here—hair spray is a basic barrier that prevents the hair from moving, whereas finishing sprays address specific problems, such as lack of shine, lack of texture, and/or volume and frizz control.

• Wax and pomade—You know how a candle burns down when you put it near a flame? Yeah—same thing will happen if you apply wax before heat styling. Melted wax in the hair = not so easy to wash out. But applied after drying, a pea-sized drop of wax or pomade warmed between the hands creates definition and piecey-ness. Great for spiking, molding, or creating übercontrol in the hair.

Better (Hair) Days Ahead

Here are the products that will give your hair a boost, restoring the volume and bounce you used to have, and giving you faith that there are better hair days ahead.

• Mousse—Because it's whipped with air and is texturally light, mousse can help not only improve hair volume, but also hold hair in place without leaving a sticky film or weighing it down. If left to air-dry, it can also help to define shape and texture. Best for fine, limp, or curly hair.

• Volumizer—Cousins to mousse, but instead of puffing hair up with foam, volumizers fill the hair shaft from the inside, causing the individual strands to swell, and then lift and support each other, giving the appearance of overall thickness. Works well for all hair types, depending on the end result you hope to achieve. Comes in many different forms such as spray, mousse, and cream.

You know how I feel—the fewer choices you have to make about your beauty routine, the better. I want to empower you with knowledge so that you can put in whatever amount of effort feels right to you, using the right products for your desired outcome so that you can get on with your life. Now it's time to select your Lazy Perfection hair care track.

Simple Track: SEAL IN MOISTURE

As soon as you get out of the shower, while your hair is still wet, you need to find a way to seal in that moisture. *This is the only step* you wash-and-go gals will need, but for the rest of us, it's a stepping-stone, a gateway to the heat styling process.

- If you have dry, frizzy hair, or hair that needs to be coaxed into submission, look for a leave-in conditioner, styling cream, or hair oil that will build a little weight to smooth and hold down strands.
- If your hair is fine or limp and you need more volume, avoid heavy oils and creams.
- If you have oily roots, apply only to the midlengths and ends of your hair.

Sophisticated Track: SEAL AND PROTECT

If you're like me and you blast your hair with insane levels of heat that occasionally result in heat tool hickeys, then applying a heat protectant is 100 percent—no, 1000 percent—essential.

Heat protectants put a barrier between your delicate follicles and the brutal heat of your dryer or iron. Think of it this way—if you put a hot iron on top of a silk shirt, it will make the fabric pucker or burn. But if you iron a silk top underneath a cotton sheet, you get the smooth result you're looking for without running the risk of damage.

Also, use the cold shot on your hair dryer. You know how when you're grilling meat you're supposed to let it rest when you take it off the heat? That's because it's still cooking as it cools down. The same thing happens with your hair, so using the cool shot stops the cooking process faster and helps prevent your hair from getting overdone.

So here are your Lazy Perfection Sophisticated Hair Steps:

- Leave-in conditioner, styling cream, or hair oil
- Heat protectant

Sexy Track: SEAL, PROTECT, AND SELECT

Ask any hairstylists, and they will almost universally tell you that the biggest issue with self-styling our hair is overapplying product. That's why the Lazy Perfection Hair Care Mantra is TWO, NOT A FEW.

A professional stylist might add a little of this and a dash of that to make you look spectacular when you walk out of the salon, but for self-styling at home, it's way too easy to go from Simple-and-Chic to Overworked-and-Sticky. Restraint is key. So look at your list of products again and decide on the look you want so you can choose the ones best for your hair —volume and shine? Smooth and frizz-free? Definition and hold?—Remember, only choose **TWO, NOT A FEW.**

To sum-up, the steps to take in the Lazy Perfection Sexy Hair Track are:

- Leave-in-conditioner, styling cream or hair oil
- Heat protectant
- A maximum of two styling products to help you achieve your desired look

And finally:

- When it comes to dry shampoo—it seems obvious, but it's important that your hair be dry when you use it and that you aim for the roots only. The absorbative properties of dry shampoo can salvage a bad hair day and be a huge time-saver when you don't wake up early enough to start from scratch, and it can even help prevent future damage by limiting the number of times per week you have to wet and heat style your hair.

But . . . those absorbtive properties can also suck away moisture from the rest of your hair, making it even more brittle and prone to breakage. A word to the wise, if the can says to shake before use, you better shake or run the risk of getting a super sticky feel at your roots.

To sum up, the steps to take in the Lazy Perfection Sexy Hair Track are:

- Leave-in-conditioner, styling cream, or hair oil
- Heat protectant
- A maximum of two styling products to help you achieve your desired look

Our hair is in a constant state of change, impacted not only by the passage of time, but also by the influences of fashion. Just remember, the best way to ensure you get on a Lazy Perfection track to looking youthful, fresh and modern is to look at your "hairstory." Revisionist history is an asset in haircare—so revise, replenish and redo!

CHAPTER TWELVE

If the Clothes Fit...

DON'T YOU ADMIRE THOSE WOMEN WHO ALWAYS LOOK SO pulled together and glamorous, even when they're wearing yoga clothes? The effortless-chic look is something TPW has down. And to top it off, her makeup always seems to work with whatever she's wearing. She's the definition of appropriate.

"Appropriate" is a tricky word in fashion. I'm not talking about "age appropriate"—I'm talking about a fashion look that's appropriate to your lifestyle, personal style, and that works in concert with your makeup and hair. Remember, everything has to go together seamlessly and in balance. You can't Nicki Minaj your face if you're Jennifer Aniston-ing your wardrobe, right? That would be pretty out of whack.

Fortunately, I have my Lazy Perfection method in place for figuring out what to wear, how to get dressed quickly, and how to do my makeup so that it all works together in a flattering, youthful, and chic way. I'm really excited to share it with you, because it's going to make your fashion choices so much more fun, flattering, and easy.

As with beauty, it's important to identify your Lazy Perfection fashion objective, and then to decide which track is the best for you—Simple, Sophisticated, or Sexy.

Feel Your Fashion

Thank goodness we live in an age when all shapes and sizes are embraced and celebrated, but most women still want a wardrobe that's going to make them look as thin as possible. It's okay to have that objective, but consider these other fashion goals:

- Do you want to look younger or more modern?
- Do you want to feel more confident?
- Do you want to express yourself in a particular way and build an image?

I think most of us Lazy Perfectionites have the same goals in mind when it comes to our fashion feelings:

- We want clothes that flatter our shape.
- We want to look current and modern—on trend, but not trendy.
- We want the colors to suit us.
- We want to be able to get dressed fast.
- We want to be appropriate for the situation and the climate.

There's that "appropriate" word again. And even though I hate being told what I can and can't wear (because I'm a wee bit rebellious at heart), the truth is that there are certain rules we need to follow, or at least take into consideration. Especially as the years go by.

Showing Some Skin

I am not ready to give up my shorts, spaghetti straps, or deep V-neck shirts. Some fashion "experts" tell you that after a certain point they're a big no-no, but I say, as long as you still feel good in them, and they are still in fashion, why not wear what you love? It's that "still in fashion" part that can trip you up.

Formulate Your Fashion

Okay. So you want to get dressed fast, feel great, and always be modern, chic, and appropriate. Sounds like it might be a tall order, but there are a few tidbits of information you can arm yourself with that will Lazy Perfectionize your process. Let's start with a good old rummage through the . . .

Pretty Skin Lost and Found

Skin and fashion go hand in hand—and pretty much all clothes reveal our skin one way or another. Showing skin can be done in a Simple, Sexy, or Sophisticated way, but, our skin changes over the years. It sucks, but it's the truth. And if we've spent our youth basking in the sun, smoking, drinking, or being otherwise bacchanalian, then our skin is prone to those changes even sooner. Sure, we all use SPF on our faces and necks, but in reality, do you know anyone who is as diligent about applying it to their décolletage, arms, or legs? Nope—me neither. Fortunately, there are ways to reclaim at least the look of youthful skin on our bodies.

- Want to wear a short skirt or short shorts but your knees are starting to get a little puckered? Pick up some light-reflective body lotion. The same way that highlighter on the face makes your skin appear smooth and dewy, light reflective lotion smooths and revitalizes the legs.

- Getting some underarm poppage when you wear sleeveless tops? A tiny and well-blended dab of waterproof foundation half a shade darker than your skin will make the protrusion look less obvious.

- Broken capillaries or spider veins getting you down? Self tanner or body bronzer is the simplest way to color-correct and camouflage.

- Want to make arms and legs as long and lean as they were when you were a gangly teen? A stripe of illuminating body sheen down the front of the shins and arms gives the illusion of length and tone.

- Hate the freckles on your décolletage? Add extra bronzer on your face to bring the tones of your face, neck, and chest in line, then blend a line of highlighter over each side of your collarbones. This draws the eyes up and away from the flat area of the chest that tends to show the signs of sun damage.
- Want to distract from other areas of your body that bother you? Show off your shoulders. Make sure to keep them exfoliated and hydrated—you can even highlight them if you want an extra glow—and they'll always be there for you to lean on when you're not feeling so great about everything else.

Look to the Lids

Pink is the new black. Navy is the new black. Black is the new black. You know what? Forget the trends when it comes to color. If it looks good on you, it looks good on you. Period.

Honestly, we can talk for hours about the way to identify whether your skin is warm or cool and what the best colors are for you to wear, but I have a way simpler Lazy Perfection trick for determining your most flattering color. It's kind of out there, but it works. Just look to your eyelids for guidance. Seriously.

Take off all your makeup and stand a little distance away from a mirror. Now, look at your eyelids. Are they the same color as the rest of your face? Congratulations—you are neutral and can wear any color under the sun. But, most women have a little discoloration on their lids, and while we fight it when it comes to applying our makeup, we can actually embrace when it comes to our fashion.

- Are your lids a little rusty red or pink? Then orange, red, and pink are your colors.
- Purple or gray? You guessed it—purple will suit you, or you can brighten up with silver.

- Deep orange or brown? Look for rich, warm colors like pumpkin, cappuccino, or bronze.

Obviously, those aren't the ONLY colors that are going to look good on you. We all need a little variety in our closets, so let's examine the full color spectrum and how you can make your makeup and apparel sing a duet in perfect harmony.

LBD, LWD, LPD . . . All the Ds

If you're anything like me, you default to black more than any other color. There's not a thing wrong with having a predominantly black wardrobe. After all, it's easy, it's slimming, it doesn't show dirt, it always looks refined, and it's a great backdrop for accessories. And—it looks good on everyone, all year round. I love the juxtaposition of a lightweight LBD in the heat of the summer—it feels a little edgier and sexier to me than the predictable coterie of bright summer colors. You just need to know how to adjust your makeup so that you look seasonally appropriate. Black in the summer requires lots of extra bronzer and warm gold, copper, or peachy tones on the cheeks and lips. That's the big secret. Not so complicated, right? It's how you can avoid looking like Winona Ryder in *Beetlejuice*.

With any color you're wearing, you have to know how to adjust your makeup so it's the most flattering. Here's what I mean.
- **Black** is the darkest of all colors, so it absorbs all the other colors around it, including those on your face. Extra blush or bronzer (or both) is crucial when you are wearing black, and an additional coat of mascara to frame your eyes will really make them "pop."
- **White** is the lightest color of all and can really brighten up your complexion . . . or totally wash it out. If you're on the fair side, bronzer will be your best friend when you're wearing white. It doesn't have

to be a lot, but a touch on your cheeks, temples, forehead, and chin won't make your skin look tan, per se, but it will make it look fresh and healthy. If you have a darker complexion, make sure to add brightness to the skin in the form of highlighter, perhaps in a sheer gold or bronze.

- Red, orange, and hot pink are what I call the heat-seeking attention-getters. In order for them to be their most flattering, all the red/pink/orange tones in your skin need to be neutralized, otherwise your face might look blotchy and overheated. Concealer and foundation are the name of the game when it comes to wearing these hotties, especially under the eyes (and on the eyelids, if necessary), around the nose, between the brows, and on the chin.

- Green, yellow, and blue are the colors of the Sirens. They tempt you like refreshing water, but if you're not careful, they can make you look seasick. It's important to make sure that you have lots of natural-looking pinks on your face when you wear these water tones, so taking care to brighten the undereye area and get a fresh flush on the cheeks with highlighter and blush will ensure that you stay afloat.

- Navy? Navy is a hero color. Everyone looks good in it because it brightens the whites of the eyes and the teeth and makes the skin look clear and fresh. An added pop of peach or rose blush and lipstick will set off the complexion even more. Navy's cousins purple, plum, and eggplant can be quite the heroes as well, by the way.

- Pastels aren't for everyone. Full stop. If you have light skin and light hair, you can get away with light pastels as long as you keep your makeup, you guessed it, light. Pastels may look chalky on deeper complexions, and the way to balance it out is to introduce the same tone into your makeup somewhere, to tie it together. A pastel lip, cheek, or shadow makes the look cohesive.

- Neutrals like buff, beige, ivory, cream, sand . . . they always just look

203

so soft and feminine and modern. The challenge comes when your face lacks the color to support your monochromatic outfit. You don't need to change the makeup you're wearing, you just need to wear more of it. Put on extra eyeliner. Add another couple of sweeps of blush. It'll wake up your whole look.

- Gray—Much like black and white, gray is a fabulous neutral. It can be dark, veering on black, or pale, veering on white, but because of the cool undertone, it's always going to make your eyes look bright and pretty. You just have to find the right shade of gray for you—lighter, cooler grays for neutral or cool complexions; darker grays for everyone else. The makeup secret with gray is to make sure you introduce at least one cool color into your makeup palette, like a slight platinum or silver sheen on your lids, a pearl highlight on your cheeks, or a slightly milky lip color. This little touch will anchor your look whereas too much warmth will sink it.

- Camel, brown, caramel . . . These warm tones are the chocolaty, delicious ones—rich and delicious. Balancing them with bronze, copper, deep pinks, and apricots will make you look as cozy and warm as a cashmere wrap.

And while we're talking about cashmere, I think we should take a moment to discuss the fashion birds and the bees.

Tex(ture)ed

That's right. The texture of your clothing can also be offset and accentuated by the makeup you wear. As with all things Lazy Perfection, it's all about balance.

- Flat, dull knit textures like suede, cashmere, wool, or bouclé can make our complexions look dull, too. Adding some strategic glow to the face is the best way to wear these fabrics. A little highlighter on the cheeks or around the tear ducts will instantly give you the look of luxury, hydration, and glow. Matte makeup with matte clothes makes for a very boring, flat look.

- High-sheen fabrics like satin, metallic, sequins, or even some leathers look glamorous and luxurious with radiant skin, lips, and eyes, particularly if you're showing lots of skin on your shoulders and décolletage. Just beware of sparkles and glitter—the addition of these chunky particles in your clothes and your makeup can take you from chic to cheap in an instant.

Now that you have a handle on how to approach your fashion colors and textures when you're applying your makeup, it's time to take a clear-eyed look at what's in your closet.

The Lazy Perfection Purge

Whether you like to shop in person at a store or online in your pajamas, the temptation to get more, more, more is always there. I'll admit that I used to be a more, more, more person . . . until I realized that Lazy Perfection not only cleared more space in my closet (and makeup kit) but it cleared more space in my brain and my schedule. You can spend the time to KonMari the hell out of your clothes, evaluating every item to see what brings you joy and then lovingly fold it and put it in its place, or you can clean things out the Lazy Perfection way, which is way faster and easier. And, your newly cleaned closet will still bring you joy!

- First, start with your shoes. They literally ground your entire fashion existence, but if they are uncomfortable—regardless of how cute they are or how expensive they were—get rid of them. Sell them on eBay, give them to a friend, donate them to charity—there's no good reason to keep shoes that hurt your feet. All those towering high heels—gone.

Booties that blister—buh-bye. Pointy-toe pumps—take a powder. I promise, after the initial shock, you won't even miss them.

- Next, look at your bras and underwear. Getting rid of the stuff that doesn't fit or flatter and replacing it with things that do will change the way your clothes look and how you feel in them. In fact, I urge you not to even look at cleaning out your clothes until you have a chance to try them on again with your girls hoisted and your panty lines eradicated.

- Then, get rid of anything that's been too small for more than three to four years. We have to be realistic about our size, and if you haven't gotten the weight off in three to four years, then chances are that if you do, by the time you do, those clothes will already be out of style. It sounds like tough love, but it's just part of the realism of Lazy Perfection.

- And your fat clothes. We all have them. For god's sake, don't get rid of them. That's something you'd regret! Just make sure that, like your skinny clothes, they're not more than a few years old and totally out of fashion. Because feeling heavy *and* unstylish is rough.

- Reevaluate what clothes to keep with a closet space:years worn ratio. Looking objectively at whether to dedicate space to your clothing is like deciding whether to break up with someone—the amount of good times you had together, divided by the amount of bad times, divided by the amount of sexy times. If the good and the sexy come out of top (wink wink), then keep on keeping on. If there's been nothing but boredom, apathy, or misery for the last little while, you've gotta cut it loose.

- Remember back in chapter 8 when I told you how many women have the same color lipstick in endless brand varieties? I'd guess the same issues arises at least a couple of times in your closet, probably with items like jeans and black pants. Approach the fashion purge the same way you did the makeup purge—don't just look at color and usefulness, look at texture and fit as well. It's no use keeping a pair of jeans that look exactly like all your other jeans . . . especially when you reach for every other pair first.

- Give yourself a fashion time line. It's a simple formula—if you haven't worn it in more than five years and you wore it less than five times, then the probability of you wearing it again is super low. It's just taking up space. Reclaim that space. Try to apply the formula to three years and three times, or two years and two times.

- Turn your accessories into décor-cessories. It's hard to part with broken jewelry or one lonely, leftover earring—they can have so much sentimental and/or monetary value. Instead of tossing it away, mount the meaningful ones in a shadow box or on a fabric. You can also do this with clothes or shoes you think are too beautiful to part with. I had a client who inherited her grandmother's extensive handbag collection, but they were too old-fashioned for her and just taking up space in her closet. We chose a couple, had them shellacked, and put them on a bookshelf. They are now adorable décor-cessories.

Sure, you can purge your clothes the same way you purge your makeup, by a process of removal and return, but clothes, shoes, and accessories take up a ton of space, and if you move it all out of your closet, where are you going to keep it? Obviously, you should fold, hang, pack, and box as much as you can so that it all looks nice and neat, but it's the hanging stuff that needs the most attention. The clothes you reach for every day should be visible, accessible, and ready-to-wear.

See Me, Feel Me, Touch Me . . .

(That's a little something for all you Who classic rock fans out there.)

When it comes to clothes, out of sight generally means out of mind. How many times have you dug around and found something only to realize: "Wow! I forgot I even had this." At the risk of sounding like the mom of teenagers that I am, mess begets mess, so if your closet isn't systematized, you're likely going to end up acquiring more stuff that you don't need, won't wear, and won't enjoy.

The way to do it is really pretty simple. You just have to follow a basic color pattern.

Into the Light

• The eye is drawn to light before dark, so grouping your clothes by color is super helpful. Start with whites, move through creams into browns, and then blue, gray, navy, black.

• Keep bright colors beside the black pieces so that you can see them "pop" against the dark background.

• If you can space things out so that there's a section for tops, skirts, pants, jackets, sweaters, and then dresses, it will help you even more. You'll know exactly where to look when you're getting dressed in a hurry.

• Suborganize by sleeve length—tank, short, long. This also helps you to find what you're looking for quickly and easily.

And now, it's time to . . .

Dress to Impress

There are some basics that every woman should have in her closet, other than workout clothes. They're the ones that set the stage for everything else, the way that good skin is the foundation for all your other makeup.

- Long, lean jeans—Skinny, straight, or boot cut, they need to fit well around the backside and thighs. Too much fabric makes your posterior look droopy (aka, Mom Jeans).
- Skinny black pants—Long or cropped, black pants are a classic that can be worn for work, special events, or casually.
- A black pencil skirt—Midknee length or just above the knee. Too short and you look too young, too long and you look too old. Knee length is juuuuust right.
- V-neck T-shirts and tops—In a variety of colors and shapes, they can be worn loose or tucked in, they draw the eye down the neck, which makes the whole body appear longer.
- A slim-fitting black jacket—Worn with jeans or a dress, it should be slightly tailored. An unstructured jacket looks too sloppy and isn't as versatile because it will never look dressed up.
- A long cardigan—It can be worn loose and slouchy over jeans, pants, or skirts or belted for a more sophisticated look.
- A little black dress—It can be dressed up or down, the number one closet must-have for all women (P.S.—Coco Chanel, the inventor of the LBD, was the epitome of Lazy Perfection!).
- Pointy-toe flats—They make the legs look longer, as though you were wearing high heels. But you can actually walk in them.
- High but comfortable shoes and sandals—You MUST be able to walk in them, and not just from the valet to the dinner table.

- **High but comfortable black booties**—Booties give the foot support in the ankle and arch so they're generally more comfortable than a regular heel, and cutting the line of the leg at the ankle draws attention to their shapeliness. Booties are a new classic, but if you prefer knee-height boots, those are great, too. Just make sure that the heel and toe shapes are still current.
- **Sporty flat shoes**—Unlike actual gym shoes, sporty shoes are a chic-er, more fashionable alternative. Gym shoes are for the gym.

The fun comes when you put your basics together and accessorize them. Fashions come and go faster with accessories than they do with clothes since they're lower-priced, smaller, and easier to manufacture. Fashion companies count on us to make impulse purchases at these lower price points, so it makes sense that they rotate new styles in and out.

Here are the classic accessories you should invest in for the long term:
- **A black tote bag and/or shoulder purse**—Suitable for work, travel, or for running around. It should be comfortable to carry and not too heavy.
- **A black, gold, or silver clutch purse**—For evenings out.
- **A large scarf**—For warmth and as an accent over a jacket, dress, or with jeans. There are hundreds of ways you can wear a scarf, à la French women who are so Lazy Perfection inspirational.
- **Gold or silver hoop earrings**—These are more interesting than studs and have more flair. Pick your size, finish, and shape based on what's most flattering for your coloring and style.
- **Stacking bracelets** in gold or silver, in a variety of shapes and sizes— The fun and versatility comes in mixing and matching them.
- **A signature piece of jewelry**—For me, it's my collection of Evil Eye

Necklaces; for you it might be a cocktail ring you wear every day, an elegant watch, or diamond earrings. Every woman should have her go-to, no-brainer jewelry that accents any outfit she's wearing, even at the gym.

And here are the "fun" trendy accessories that come in and out of fashion where you don't need to spend a lot to get a lot of look:

- **Sunglasses** (although they should be UVA/UVB protective at the very least)
- **Statement jewelry**—Gold/silver/gems in larger pieces—cha-ching! Faux and cocktail jewelry is every bit as chic, and you can afford to get more of it!
- **Hats**—Unless you're really a hat person or live at the beach, there's just no reason to spend a lot.
- **Statement handbags**—All the bells and whistles time-stamp your purse in a specific year and can look dated fast.
- **Runway-, celebrity-, or editorial-inspired clothing**—The second they're over, they are OVER. Get them, wear them, enjoy them, then move them along.
- **Trendy shoes**, like platforms, T-straps, gladiator sandals—The most you can expect to get out of a trend in shoes is three years before they start to look dated.
- **Valet parking shoes**—They're too high to wear for more than twenty steps, but damn they're hard to resist. No need to spend a fortune here, but by all means, go for it!

Lazy and Lovely

Now, I am not going to talk about "athleisure" apparel here. I have been known to indulge in all-day yoga pants from time to time, but it's more straight-up "lazy" than Lazy Perfection. As you know from the beauty chapters, Lazy Perfection isn't about making *no* effort, it's about making the right effort and choosing the details that will be simple but significant for you.

Simple

This is for the mom who is going to a PTO meeting, having lunch with a friend, going to a school performance; or for the weekends when you have no professional obligations but want to appear put together; or for running errands.

- Skinny jeans or skinny black pants, cropped if it suits
- V-neck or low-buttoned blouse, half-tucked in the front to give some shape at the waist
- A trendy purse
- Sporty shoes
- Your signature jewelry

Sophisticated

This is for anyone who has to go to an office, meet with clients, have lunch with friends or colleagues, go on a date, go to a casual event, or who just wants to feel a little more dressed up.

- Skinny black pants or pencil skirt
- Pointy-toe flats (with skirt or cropped pants—not with long pants) or booties
- Deep V-neck top, tucked in to appear tailored but softly bloused over

- Slim jacket (if the weather is cool)
- Shoulder or tote purse
- Scarf wrapped over jacket or tied to handle of tote purse (if the weather is cool)
- Stacking bangles
- Hoop earrings
- Signature jewelry

Sexy

Va-Va-Voom. You are hitting the town, have a hot date, or just feel like getting all dolled up.
- Black dress or pencil skirt with deep-V top (extra deep, please)
- Booties, high sandals, or sexy heels
- Clutch purse or trend purse
- Statement jewelry
- Signature jewelry
- *ATTITUDE . . .*

That's right, Lazy Perfection lovelies . . . it's about the attitude. It's about doing your hair, putting on your makeup, and getting out the door feeling put together, chic, and confident—without having to spend a lot of time doing it.

Well it seems my job here is done. You've learned everything I can teach out about how to choose your customized Lazy Perfection Track for all facets of your life—your physical features, your technical makeup skills, your lifestyle, and your personal style.

My hope for you, and for all Lazy Perfectionites, is that you will go off into the world feeling a little brighter, a little chic-er, and a little less stressed about your beauty routine. So next time you're in a Starbucks at 7:00 a.m. with well-concealed dark spots and soft, shiny lips, look for me. I'll be the one hiding behind my sunglasses, thinking to myself to how effortless you look. Congratulations, Lazy Perfectionite. You are officially a TPW.

Acknowledgments

MY HUSBAND AND DAUGHTERS CAN PROBABLY COUNT ON one hand the number of home-cooked meals they've had since I started to work on this book. Doug, Lila, Phoebe, and Olivia—thank you for bearing with me as I struggled through the process of this enormous project and for keeping your senses of humor even when mine vanished. I am immensely blessed to have a happy, healthy, devoted, and loving family.

Thank you to Jim Karas who is responsible for putting me on the path not just to my fabulous PR team, but to the incredibly talented and knowledgeable Nancy Hancock, without whom this process *truly* would never have happened. Nancy—the insights you shared, the work you put in, the smart—and tough—questions you asked, your patience and positive attitude, and your complete faith in Lazy Perfection has brought me much comfort, and I am fully aware that I owe this entire experience to you.

To my fabulous assistant/graphic designer/account executive/office renaissance man, Leina Kameyama. You have kept the Lazy Perfection fires burning during these last many months and enabled me to focus on this project, all while being more chic and Lazy Perfection than anyone I know. Thank you from the bottom of my heart.

To my literary agent Yfat Reiss Gendell at Foundry, many thanks to you for seeing the value in Lazy Perfection right off the bat, and for having confidence that when it comes to their beauty rituals, women want not just simplicity, but education. And thank you for bringing Jennifer Kasius and Running Press into my life. Jennifer, you have been such a collaborative partner, and I thank you for being receptive and open to my ideas.

Kelly Davis, Dakota Isaacs, Samantha Trenk, and Jenny Lin (and Sasha Goldfarb) at KFDPR—you're the dream team and I couldn't love you ladies more. Eric Himel—fashion stylist extraordinaire and BFF for almost three decades—for being my sounding board, punching bag, and fashion consultant, thank you is not enough.

The amazing team at Joyus, and all the fabulous producers and editors who have been so patient and lit me so well—bless you all.

Lily Garfield, Nicky Kinnaird, Cecil Booth, Laura Kofoid, Liz Scott, Justin Smith, Chris Hobson, Nathaniel Hawkins, Troy Surratt, and Marc Landsberg—thank you for all your sage counsel. Dr. Keren Horn, I am proud to call you not just my doctor, but my friend, and I am so grateful for you. Dr. Carolyn Jacob—thank you for always being so gracious and available.

The health experts who keep me limber, strong, and motivated— Ryan Doody and Lisa Miranda—thank you for providing me with the foundation of good physical stamina, and huge thanks to my team of beauty peeps who smooth away the rough edges and keep me looking fresh and shiny—Cynthia Davila, Erin DeVita, Anthony Cristiano, Darrin Goins, and Becky Wolter-Janopoulos, and my home team of Maria DeLao, Kathleen Bertuca, and Katie Blehart for always being there to help us pick up the pieces.

I am totally blessed to be surrounded by a coterie of smart, successful, funny, supportive friends, and by parents, siblings, in-laws, and nieces/ nephews I completely, totally adore. My life is better for having all of you in it.

And so, in conclusion, and to sum up . . . writing a book is not Lazy Perfection.

Product Recommendations

CONCEALER	LUXURY	PRESTIGE/INDIE	MASS	CLEAN
Concealer - Cream	Dolce & Gabbana Perfect Matte Concealer	Amazing Cosmetics Hydrate Concealer	Maybelline Facestudio Master Conceal	Well People Bio Correct
Concealer - Click Pen	La Prairie Light Fantastic Cellular Concealing Brightening Eye Treatment	ByTerry Touche Veloutee Highlighting Concealer	Physicians Formula Super CCC Correct + Conceal + Cover	Beautycounter Touchup Skin Concealer Pen
Concealer - Stick/Pan	Cle de Peau Beaute Concealer Correctuer Visage	Benefit Fake Up Hydrating Under Eye Concealer	Revlon PhotoReady Concealer	NuEvolution Camouflage Cream
FOUNDATION				
Primer	Guerlain Meteorites Base Perfecting Pearls	Hourglass Veil Mineral Primer	Almay Smart Shade CC Luminous Primer	Juice Beauty Phyto-Pigments Illuminating Primer
Foundation - Light Coverage (Tinted Moisturizer, BB or CC Cream)	Chanel Vitalumiere Aqua	It Cosmetics CC Cream	Boots No7 Dual Action Tinted Moisturizer	MD Solar Sciences Mineral Beatuy Balm Broad Spectrum SPF 50
Foundation - Medium Coverage	Giorgio Armani Luminous Silk Foundation	Nars All Day Luminous Weightless Foundation	L'Oreal True Match Lumi Healthy Luminous Makeup	Vapour Atmosphere Soft Focus Foundation
Foundation - Full Coverage	Charlotte Tilbury Magic Foundation	Clinique Beyond Perfecting Foundation	Maybelline Dream Velvet	NuEvolution Complete Coverage
Foundation - Oil Free/ Matte	Chanel Velvet Lumiere	Too Faced Born This Way	Maybelline Fit Me Matte	RMS Beauty Uncover Up
Foundation - Powder	Serge Lutens Compact Foundation	Lancome Dual Finish Foundation	NYX Powder Stay Matte	W3ll People Altruist Powder
Foundation - Stick	Tom Ford Traceless Foundation Stick	Anastasia Beverly Hills Stick Foundation	Maybelline Fit Me Shine Free + Balance Foundation	W3ll People Narcissist Foundation Stick
Bronzer - Satin Powder	Guerlain Terracotta Light Bronzing Powder	Hourglass Ambient Lighting Bronzer	Physician's Formula Bronze Booster	Studio78 Paris We Evade Bronzing Powder
Bronzer - Matte Powder	Chantecaille Compact Soleil Bronzer	Bobbi Brown Bronzing Powder	NYX Matte Bronzer	Han Skincare Cosmetics Bronzer
Bronzer - Cream/Liquid	Giorgio Armani Maestro Liquid Bronzer	Bare Minerals Sheer Sun Serum Bronzer	Sonia Kashuk Undetectable Cream Bronzer	W3ll People Bio Bronzer Stick
Highlighter - Powder	Dior Diorskin Nude Air Luminizer Powder	Kevyn Aucoin Candlelight Powder	Physician's Formula Mineral Glow Pearls	Lily Lolo Illuminator
Highlighter - Cream/ Liquid	Tom Ford Skin Illuminator	Clinique Chubby Stick Sculpting Highlight	Flower Glisten Up	Tata Harper Illuminator

FOUNDATION	LUXURY	PRESTIGE/INDIE	MASS	CLEAN
Contour - Powder	Chanel Les Beiges Healthy Glow Sheer Color	Kevyn Aucoin The Sculpting Powder	Fiona Stiles Sheer Sculpting Palette	Lily Lolo Contour Duo
Contour - Cream	Tom Ford Shade and Illuminate	Burberry Beauty Face Contour Stick	Sonia Kashuk Chic Defining Contour Stick	Tata Harper Very Bronzing
Powder - Setting	Charlotte Tilbury Airbrush Flawless Finish Powder	RCMA Makeup No Color Powder	Palladio Rice Powder	RMS Beauty Un-Powder
BLUSH				
Powder Blush	Givenchy Le Prisme Powder Blush	Laura Mercier Second Skin Cheek Color	Cover Girl TruBlend Blush	Lily Lolo Mineral Blush
Cream Blush	Le Metiers de Beaute Crème Fresh Tint	It Cosmetics Bye Bye Lines Serum	NYX Rouge Crème Blush	Kjaer Weis Cream Blush
Stain	Chantecaille Cheek Gelee	Benefit Benetint	Sonia Kashulk Lip and Cheek Tint	Vapour Aura Multi-Stain
Cream to Powder	Chanel Le Blush Crème de Chanel	Benefit Majorette	Maybelline Dream Bouncy	Jane Iredale In Touch Cream Blush
Gel/Mousse	ByTerry Blush Glace	Laura Geller Air Whipped Blush	L'Oreal Visible Lift Blur Blush	Josie Maran Coconut Water Cheek Gelee
Liquid/Serum	Giorgio Armani Maestro Fusion Blush	Perricone MD No Blush Blush	e.l.f Studio HD Blush	Milk Makeup Blush Oil
EYES/MASCARA/ LASH CURLERS				
Lid Primer	By Terry Hyaluronic Eye Primer	Nars Pro Prime	Milani Eyeshadow Primer	Lily Lolo Prime Focus Eyelid Primer
Eyeshadow	Tom Ford Eye Quad	Surratt Beauty Artistique Eyeshadow	Wet 'n Wild Eyeshadow	RMS Swift Powder Eyeshadow
Eyeshadow Stick	ByTerry Ombre Blackstar Cream Eyeshadow	Burberry Beauty Eye Colour Contour	Rimmel Scandaleyes Eyeshadow Stick	Vapour Beauty Mezmerize Eye Color Classic
Eyeliner	Chanel Les Yeux Waterproof Stylo	Urban Decay 24/7 Glide On Eye Pencil	L'Oreal Pencil Perfect Eyeliner	W3ll People Hypnotist Eye Pencil
Mascara - Volume	Charlotte Tilbury Legendary Lashes	Urban Decay Perversion Mascara	Maybelline Full 'n Soft Mascara	Dr. Hauschka Volume Mascara
Mascara - Length	Dolce & Gabbana Secret Eyes Mascara	Peter Thomas Roth Lashes to Die for Mascara	Physician's Formula Eye Booster Mascara	Kjaer Weis Mascara
Eyelash Curler - Regular	Cle de Peau	Kevyn Aucoin	e.l.f. Lash Curler	n/a
Eyelash Curler - Deepset or Monolid	Shiseido	Surratt Beauty	Tweezerman Pro Master Lash Curler	n/a

LIPS	LUXURY	PRESTIGE/INDIE	MASS	CLEAN
Lipstick - Cream	Tom Ford Lip Color	Laura Mercier Crème Smooth Lip Color	L'Oreal Paris Color Riche Lipstick	Vapour Siren Lipstick
Lipstick - Velvet	YSL Rouge Pur Couture	Nars Velvet Matte Lip Pencil	Burt's Bee's Lipstick	Kjaer Weis Lipstick
Lipstick - Satin	Guerlain Rouge G	Edward Bess Ultra Slick Lipstick	e.l.f. Moisturizing Lipstick	Juice Beauty Satin Lip Cream
Lipstick - Balm/Sheer	Chanel Rouge Coco Shine	Becca Sheer Tint	Cover Girl Baby Lips	Ilia Tinted Lip Conditioner
Lipstick - Stain/Long Wear	Serge Lutens Water Lip Color	Hourglass Opaque Rouge Liquid Lipstick	Maybelline Super Stay 24	Juice Beauty Liquid Lip Stain
Lipgloss	Chantecaille Brilliant Gloss	Nars Larger Than Life Lipgloss	NYX Butter Gloss	Lily Lolo Natural Lip Gloss
Lip Pencil - Skinny	Charlotte Tilbury Lip Cheat	Urban Decay 24/7 Glide On Lip Pencil	NYX Slim Lip Pencil	Lily Lolo Natural Lip Pencil
Lip Pencil - Chubby	Sisley Paris Phyto Lip Twist	Nars Satin Lip Pencil	Revlon Matte Balm	Juice Beauty Luminous Lip Crayon
BROWS				
Brow Pencil	Tom Ford Eyebrow Sculptor	Hourglass Arch Brow Sculpting Pencil	NYX Microbrow	Alima Pure Eyebrow Pencil
Brow Pencil Fine Tip	Dior Diorshow Brow Styler	Surratt Beauty Expressioniste Brow Pencil	Maybelline Eye Studio Master Precise	Jane Iredale Retractable Brow Pencil
Brow Powder	Tom Ford Brow Sculpting Kit	Anastasia Beverly Hills Brow Powder Duo	Flower Beauty Take a Brow Complete Brow Kit	Peek Beauty Natural Stain Brow Powder
Brow Cream (potted)	Armani Eye and Brow	Laura Mercier Brow Definer	Milani Stay Put Brow Color	Ecobrow
Brow Gel - Clear	Chantecaille Perfecting Gel	Surratt Beauty Brow Pomade	Ardell Brow Sculpting Gel	Bloom Brow Gel
Brow Gel - Tinted	Dior Brow Styler Gel	Glossier Boy Brow	L'Oreal Tinted Brow Gel	Wunderbrow
TOOLS				
Makeup Brushes	Tom Ford	Jenny Patinkin	Real Techniques	Sigma
Makeup Sponge	ByTerry Sponge Foundation Brush	Beauty Blender	Real Techniques	Jane Iredale Flocked Sponge

BODY MAKEUP	LUXURY	PRESTIGE/INDIE	MASS	CLEAN
Waterproof Foundation	Estee Lauder Double Wear Maximum Cover Camouflage	MAC Face and Body	Miracle Skin Transformer Body SPF 20	Jane Iredale Dream Tint
Wash Off Bronzer	Charlotte Tilbury Super-model Body	Scott Barnes Body Bling	NYX Born to Glow Liquid Illuminator	Josie Maran Argan Illuminizer
Illuminating Body Cream	Lancer Dani Glowing Skin Perfector	Perfekt Liquid Gold Illumiating Perfector	Olay Quench Shimmer	Pretty Peaushun
SKINCARE				
Facewash	Cle de Peau Clarifying Cleansing Foam	Fresh Soy Milk Cleanser	Cetaphil	Goop Luminous Melting Cleanser
Multi-Serum	La Prairie Anti-Aging Rapid Response Booster	It Cosmetics Bye Bye Lines Serum	Hylamide SubQ Anti-Age Serum	Tata Harper Rejuventaing Serum
AHA Exfoliant	ReVive Glycolic Renewal Peel System	Ren Skincare Glycolic Lactic Radiance Renewal Mask	Pixi Glow Tonic	Tammy Fender Epi Peel
BHA Treatment	Erno Laszlo Anti-Blemish Beta Wash	Paula's Choice BHA Skin Perfecting Liquid	Aveeno Clear Complex-ion Foaming Cleanser	Herbivore Botanicals Blue Tansy Mask
Antioxidant Serum	Natura Bisse C+C Vitamin Complex	Sarah Chapman Skinesis Age Repair Concentrate	Boots No.7 Protect and Perfect Serum	Marie Veronique C, E and Ferulic Acid
Retinoid	111 Skin Celestial Black Diamond Retinol Oil	Golfaden MD Wake Up Call	ROC Retinol Correction Night Cream	Marie Veronique Gentle Retinol Night Serum
Moisturizer	Crème de la Mer	Kate Somerville Instant Rewind	Neutrogena Hydro Boost Water Gel	Theraphi Rose Otto Honey Moisturizer
Eye Cream	Sisley Supremeya Eyes at Night	Kate Somerville Line Release Eye Cream	Oil of Olay Total Effects Anti-Aging Eye Treatment	Goop Perfecting Eye Cream
Neck Cream	Estee Lauder Resilience Lift Firming/Sculpting	Cellex-C Advanced C Neck Firming Cream	L'Oreal Paris Age Perfect Hydra Nutrition Golden Balm	Skin Owl Neck + Super Smoothing and Contouring Neck Concentrate
Growth Factors	Erno Lazslo Firmarine Lift Serum	Neocutis Bio-Serum Intensive Treatment	Osmosis Pur Medical Skincare Mist	Acure Organics Night Cream
SPF	Chantecaille Ultra Sun Protection 45	Elta MD UV Daily 40	La Roche Posay Anthelios	MD Solar Sciences
Tinted SPF	Clarins UV Plus Anti-Pollution SPF 50	MD Solar Sciences Mineral Tinted Cream	Almay Smart Shade CC Cream SPF 35	Suntegrity 5-in-1 Tinted Moisturizer Sunscreen
Hand Cream	Amore Pacific Time Response Intensive Hand Renewal Cream	Dermelect Timeless Anti-Aging Hand Treatment	Hand Chemistry	Pai Skincare Fragonia & Sea Buckthorn Instant Therapy Hand Cream
Lip Balm/Treatment	La Mer The Lip Balm	VenEffect Anti-Aging Lip Treatment	Aquaphor	RMS Beauty Lip and Skin Balm

Index

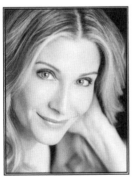

JENNY PATINKIN is a prominent makeup artist, beauty expert, and entrepreneur. The founder of Lazy Perfection Beauty School, Jenny is known for her simple, unfussy approach to beauty. She appears regularly on network TV and prominent digital media channels, is a beloved on-air host for Joyus.com, and her expert advice and makeup artistry are frequently featured in publications such as *Martha Stewart Living, Real Simple, Health,* and *Bridal Guide,* among many others. Jenny's Lazy Perfection makeup brushes are sold in luxury boutiques across the country. Visit her at jennypatinkin.com.